Nursing Ethics

Jones and Bartlett Books on Ethics and Related Titles of Interest

The Abortion Controversy: A Reader
Louis P. Pojman, The University of Mississippi and
Francis Beckwith, University of Nevada Las Vegas, Editors

Bioethics: A Committee Approach, Brendan Minogue, Youngstown State University

Cross-Cultural Perspectives in Medical Ethics: Readings
Robert M. Veatch, The Kennedy Institute of Ethics, Georgetown University, Editor

Ethics Consultation
John LaPuma, Center for Clinical Ethics, Lutheran General Hospital,
Park Ridge, Illinois and
David Schiedermayer, Department of Medicine, Medical College of Wisconsin,
Milwaukee, Wisconsin

Health Assessment in Nursing Practice, Third Edition
Jorge Grimes, SUNY Health Science Center, Syracuse and
Elizabeth Burns, Niagra University

Life and Death: A Reader in Moral Problems
Louis P. Pojman, The University of Mississippi, Editor

Life and Death: Grappling with the Moral Dilemmas of Our Time
Louis P. Pojman, The University of Mississippi

Medical Ethics, Second Edition
Robert M. Veatch, The Kennedy Institute of Ethics, Georgetown University, Editor

Moral Theory: A Contemporary Overview
Joseph P. DeMarco, Cleveland State University

Nursing Ethics: Therapeutic Caring Presence
Anne H. Bishop and John R. Scudder, Jr., Lynchburg College

Perspectives on Death and Dying
Gere B. Fulton and Eileen K. Metress, University of Toledo

Nursing Ethics
Therapeutic Caring Presence

Anne H. Bishop
John R. Scudder, Jr.

Lynchburg College

Jones and Bartlett Publishers
Sudbury, Massachusetts

Boston   London   Singapore

Editorial, Sales, and Customer Service Offices
Jones and Bartlett Publishers
One Exeter Plaza
Boston, MA 02116
1-800-832-0034
617-859-3900

Jones and Bartlett Publishers International
7 Melrose Terrace
London W6 7RL
England

Library of Congress Cataloging-in-Publication Data

Bishop, Anne H., 1935–
    Nursing ethics : therapeutic caring presence / Anne Bishop, John R. Scudder, Jr.
       p. cm. -- (Jones and Bartlett series in philosophy)
    Includes bibliographical references and index.
    ISBN 0-86720-969-0
     1. Nursing ethics.   I. Scudder, John R., 1926– . II. Series.
RT85.B57 1996
    174'.2 --dc20
                                    95-32768
                                        CIP

Acquisitions Editors: Arthur C. Bartlett and Nancy E. Bartlett
Production Administrator: Anne S. Noonan
Manufacturing Buyer: Dana L. Cerrito
Editorial Production Service: Book 1
Typesetting: Seahorse Prepress/Book 1
Printing and Binding: Braun-Brunfield, Inc.
Cover Design: Joyce Weston
Cover Printing: New England Book Components, Inc.

Printed in the United States of America
99 98 97 96 95   10 9 8 7 6 5 4 3 2 1

Contents

Foreword

A little over thirty years ago, philosophers began to become directly involved with the health professions. Their efforts focused primarily on ethics, and these in turn almost exclusively concerned medicine: physicians, not nurses, were the focal point; the physician-patient relationship, not that between nurses and patients, held the limelight. Not surprisingly, within that focus, philosophers concerned with ethics tended to be more captivated by the publicly-prominent topics of the day than by the actual practices of physicians; much of their agenda, as it were, was (and in many ways continues to be) set by the media. The table of contents of practically any "textbook" tells the story:[1] abortion, definition of death, organ transplantation, do-not-resuscitate orders, withdrawing and withholding life supports, living will, distributing scarce resources, human experimentation, and the like.

To learn about "ethics and health care" was to learn primarily about the sorts of problems that confronted physicians—and, of course, patients—for the most part in acute-care, *crisis* situations. Philosophers, of course, were not seen (perhaps with greater wisdom than was realized) as decision makers (decisions belong to doctors and patients); at best, philosophers could perform "ethical analyses" and perhaps make recommendations based upon them. Ethical analysis, furthermore, was mostly thought to be a matter of "applying" certain "principles" and "rules" (both taken as already at hand) to practical situations. But as there are many different ethical theories and principles at hand that are at odds with each other,[2] doctors reasonably asked "ethicists" which of the theories was the "right" one—a question at once decidedly uncomfortable (hardly settled within the hallowed halls of philosophy) and impossible to answer (presuming, as it does, a point of view enjoyed by no mere human).

For all the difficulties, nevertheless, one approach quickly won wide favor. With "human rights" increasingly endorsed, it was accepted that one particular principle was basic—a principle derived in substantial part from legal cases in the 1950s and 1960s, and from public discussions centered around questions of human experimentation (which highlighted such options as "informed consent" and "confidentiality"). This principle was *autonomy*, the "right of self-determination." On the other hand, it was also noted that physicians were by tradition, and often by inclination, guided by two principles apparently different from autonomy: helping patients—*beneficence*—and, if unable to help them, then doing them no harm—*nonmaleficence*. The real question, then, was now to balance the patient's autonomy with the doctor's responsibility short of falling into a kind of relativism or even anarchy (where too much autonomy leads), or on the other hand into an unfortunate arrogance (paternalism that results from too much stress on the doctor's beneficence). Since medical care in our times requires equitable management of scarce resources, *justice* also came to play a prominent role.[3] The work of ethics thus came to mean little more than applying these principles to the facts of any case.[4]

If anything, nurses were, like social workers and other health professionals, left to their own devices—including attending to questions of ethics. Even here, however, learning about ethics most often meant encountering the same ideas found in the bulk of the ethics (not inaccurately termed "medical ethics") literature: autonomy, beneficence, nonmaleficence, justice. If a nurse wanted to know about ethics, the thing to do was to ask the "expert," a person well-schooled in ethics—which commonly meant a philosopher who, of course, pretty much advocated the same line as was already well accepted. What passed for "nursing ethics" thus differed but slightly from "medical ethics"—despite the fact that most nurses had considerable difficulty seeing themselves as in the midst of "ethical issues" only when in a "crisis" of the sort found in the burgeoning ethics literature. Both "medical" and "nursing" ethics, as well as the ethics governing other health professionals (and, presumably, patients and families, though these were only rarely analyzed as such[5]) were thus regarded as a matter of the application of ethical theories already on hand—one in particular taking precedence: autonomy. Philosophers analyzed, physicians applied. Nurses and the other health professionals for the most part looked on, according to what critical action was taking place, and where.

This view of nursing began to be challenged from within nursing itself, with Sally Gadow (also a philosopher),[6] Patricia Benner,[7] and Bishop and Scudder (the latter a philosopher)[8] [9] leading the way and basing much of their thinking on and in response to the feminist ethics of Nell Noddings[10] and Carol Gilligan.[11] They brought a quite "different voice" to bear on questions of ethics and health care, especially regarding the role of nurses in caring for patients. They, and growing numbers of other nurses (and a few philosophers), exhibited not only a well-honed critical discontent with the accepted "principlist" view,[12] but also a keen sense that developing a sound idea of *nursing* ethics requires being specially attentive and responsive to the particularities and circumstances of actual nursing practices (an insight that other writers on ethics were bringing to bear on medicine as well[13]).

The several writings by Anne Bishop and Jack Scudder have been at the forefront of both the criticism and the attention to nursing and to the "ethics" that is firmly and integrally embedded in its practices. In their earlier works, they were not, however, specifically concerned with developing that "ethics," believing that they needed first of all to be as clear as possible about the nature and character of nursing practice. Nurses, perhaps uniquely, practice "in-between" patients and doctors, patients and family members, chaplains and doctors, often in-between nurses and doctors and even doctors and doctors. At the same time, their practice brings them in direct, wholly intimate contact with patients—the subjects of their most immediate concern—through touching, talking, feeling, and listening. Nurses' actions are designed to comfort, ease, calm, encourage, and assist in order to, as Bishop and Scudder insist in the present study, "foster the well-being of others" (p. 15). In this "way of being [that] fosters trust, mutual concern, and positive attitudes that promote good health" (p. 65), is a key insight that guides their approach to the ethics of nursing: it is a profession, to be sure, but here the "profession does not establish the moral sense. The moral sense establishes the profession" (p. 140)—a point that could well be made about any of the health professions. In their new work, there is not only a continuation of their earlier insights and directions, but quite clearly a distinct and important advance in our understanding of ethics: the incisive way in which major philosophical—but pre-eminently practical—insights are discovered within the wholly concrete life of nursing practice. Careful attention to their unfolding arguments makes very clear that no one profession could possibly have a lock on what ethics is all about.

Their practical, interpretive effort to disclose the ethical character of nursing requires careful attention be paid to its practice. By doing so, Bishop and Scudder continue and advance their fascinating and thoughtful voyage into one of the most concrete and distinctive regions of human life: the intimate, complex relationships among sick people and those who both care for them and seek to take care of them. It is a study that is most rewarding for its important insights into and understanding of ethics in its broader, if still deeply troubled, presence in our society.

—*Richard M. Zaner, Vanderbilt University Medical Center*

References

1. For instance, Ronald Munson, *Intervention and Reflection: Basic Issues in Medical Ethics*, Belmont, CA: Wadsworth, Inc. 4th edition, 1992, hardly has a word about nurses or their "ethics."
2. Alasdair MacIntyre, *After Virtue*, Notre Dame, IN: University of Notre Dame Press, 1982.
3. Albert R. Jonsen, Mark Siegler, William J. Winslade, *Clinical Ethics*, New York: McGraw-Hill, 1992.
4. Tom L. Beauchamp and James J. Childress, *Principles of Biomedical Ethics*, New York: Oxford University Press, 4th edition, 1994.
5. A notable exception is an anthology edited by Anne H. Bishop and John R. Scudder, Jr.: *Caring, Curing, Coping: Nurse, Physician, Patient, Relationships*, University, AL: University of Alabama Press, 1985.
6. Sally Gadow, "Existential Advocacy: Philosophical Foundation of Nursing," in S. Spicker and S. Gadow (eds.), *Nursing: Images and Ideals: Opening Dialogue with the Humanities*, New York: Springer, 1980.
7. Patricia Benner, *From Novice to Expert: Excellence and Power in Clinical Nursing Practice*, Menlo Park, CA: Addison-Wesley, 1984.
8. Anne H. Bishop and John R. Scudder, Jr., *The Practical, Moral, and Personal Sense of Nursing: A Phenomenological Philosophy of Practice*, Cf. p. 227 Albany, NY: State University of New York Press, 1990.
9. Anne H. Bishop and John R. Scudder, Jr., *Nursing: The Practice of Caring*, New York: The National League for Nursing Press, 1991.
10. Nel Noddings, *Caring: A Feminine Approach to Ethics and Moral Education*, Berkeley, CA: University of California Press, 1984.
11. Carol Gilligan, *In A Different Voice: Psychological Theory and Women's Development*, Cambridge, MA: Harvard University Press, 1982.
12. E. R. DuBose, R. Hamel and L. J. O'Connell (eds.), *A Matter of Principles? Ferment in U.S. Bioethics*, The Park Ridge Center for the Study of Health, Faith and Ethics, Valley Forge, PA: Trinity Press International, 1994.
13. Richard M. Zaner, *Ethics and the Clinical Encounter*, Englewood Cliffs, NJ: Prentice Hall, 1988.

Preface

Richard Zaner, in his foreword, gives a perceptive account of the development of health care ethics that sets the ethical context for this book. Although that development, and specifically Zaner's ethics, has contributed to our interpretation of nursing ethics, our treatment of the subject grew out of our phenomenological investigation of the meaning of nursing. From examining nursing as it is practiced, we interpreted nursing as the practice of caring. Because nursing, like all practices, has a dominant moral sense and caring itself is a moral activity, nursing ethics is inherent in nursing practice.

Nursing ethics concerns articulating the moral sense of nursing and appraising how it is fulfilled, rather than applying ethical theories to nursing practice. The moral sense of nursing is fulfilled through the caring presence of nurses that achieves the therapeutic intent of nursing practice. This interpretation of nursing practice requires that nursing ethics begin with and stick with the moral sense of nursing. When the moral sense of nursing is realized, nursing ethics becomes engaged in nursing practice itself. The moral sense of practice, not ethical theory, is the driving force of nursing ethics.

We are grateful to many people for helping us develop and publish this book. Over the years we have shared works in progress with Richard Zaner and Patricia Benner for their critical appraisal and dialogical response. Zaner has long contributed to our interpretations of health care and of ethics. We owe to him the suggestion that we conclude the book with a dialogue concerning the meaning of nursing ethics as we each have come to understand it. Benner, who has contributed substantially to our previous work, has applied her penetrating criticism and productive suggestions to this work.

In Robert Ginsberg we found an editor with a kindred spirit, one who made suggestions to free us from the stuffy language that plagues those of us who learned to write in the academy. His deep sensitivity to what we are doing encouraged us to be creative in tone and language, as well as in content. In Arthur C. Bartlett we found a publisher with a congenial spirit who made himself available to assist our project. Ginsberg and Bartlett made the complicated task of getting this book into print a pleasant and meaningful experience. Others who contributed critically or editorially to our work are Nancy E. Bartlett, Anne Noonan, Wanda Teays, Peter Appleby, Betty Ferrell, and Brendan Minogue.

For their encouragement, patience, and support during the research, writing, and preparation of this book, we are pleased to thank—once again—our spouses, Mary and Bobby.

Anne H. Bishop
John R. Scudder, Jr.

1

Why Another Book
on Nursing Ethics?

Nursing is engaged in an exciting rediscovery of its meaning as a caring practice. This new venture calls for a nursing ethics that takes seriously the meaning inherent in nursing practice. Nursing traditionally assumed that it was a caring practice, but that assumption was never adequately articulated, nor was its meaning thought out. The current reinterpretation of nursing is focused on recovering the initial meaning of nursing as a caring practice but in a way that discloses the deeper meaning of nursing practice. We have taken part in this development by interpreting nursing first as a practice with an inherent moral sense (Bishop and Scudder 1990) and then as the practice of caring that fulfills that moral sense (Bishop and Scudder 1991).

We believe that nursing needs to develop its own ethics focused on nursing practice and the fulfillment of its moral sense, rather than on the application of philosophical ethics. In taking this position, we are not denying the important contribution that applied ethics has made and is making to nurses in facing moral dilemmas. Instead, we are advocating a new approach to nursing ethics that speaks directly to the situation of practicing nurses by taking seriously the moral intent of nursing practice.

This book on ethics is a continuation of our previous work, which has attempted to make sense out of nursing in a way that helps nurses become better nurses. We have contended that nursing is a practice with an inherent moral sense. Nursing is neither a theoretical activity nor a practical activity in the sense of being limited to the "tricks of the trade." Nursing does not begin with theory that is applied to the world to achieve certain ends. Instead, it is a practice, in that it is made up of practical ways of fostering the good, that is, the well-being of persons. Although it is a practice, it is not practical in the limited sense that it was earlier in this century. Then, nursing was taught primarily as techniques and procedures that had to be followed precisely, with little attention to the context of meaning. As nursing developed, an attempt was made to supply the context of meaning from nursing theories drawn from outside nursing. Although we have been critical of this approach to nursing in our books, these nursing theories did move nursing beyond techniques and procedures. Unfortunately, these theories not only moved thought about nursing away from practice but also moved it away from the moral sense in which that practice is rooted. And it is that moral sense that has to be at the root of any nursing ethics.

We will attempt to develop a nursing ethics that is rooted in the moral sense of practice. This approach is different from the typical biomedical approach, in which ethical issues are generally considered to result from advances in modern technology. The biomedical ethics approach implies that medicine, and perhaps nursing, is a technological activity that occasionally spawns moral problems that require the help of experts called ethicists. These experts usually apply ethics to nursing problems by converting nursing problems into ethical issues as formulated by philosophers. Practical problems and dilemmas taken from practice are often used to illustrate how to employ philosophical norms and reasoning, rather than how to achieve the good at which the practice aims. Books on medical and nursing ethics are replete with such examples. Usually, they are carefully selected to illustrate the importance of applied ethics and the use of philosophical norms and reasoning to resolve moral problems in health care.

In the applied approach, the stress is usually on whether the action taken coheres with ethical principles, such as autonomy or utilitarianism, rather than on fostering the well-being of the patient. Thus, ethics is primarily concerned with taking action that conforms to an ethical principle, rather than with being therapeutic by fostering the well-being of patients. Nursing needs an approach to ethics that takes seriously the moral sense of nursing and thus speaks directly to practitioners.

It was this insight that initially led us to write this book. The stress on the moral sense of nursing was so pronounced in one of our earlier books that it was twice reviewed as a book on nursing ethics. That book was not a book on nursing ethics; it was a book that showed that nursing was a practice with an inherent moral sense. Rather than developing an ethics of nursing, we merely argued that any nursing ethics had to be rooted in that moral sense.

This book is an attempt to develop a nursing ethics that is rooted in the moral sense of nursing. Chapter 2 deals with nursing as an ethics of practice in which the motivation to care and the practice of care are integrally related. In Chapter 3, we describe, illustrate, and articulate the caring presence that is an essential aspect of any caring ethics in nursing. Although we originally intended to write this book on caring presence, we discovered that caring presence, even when predicated on the moral sense of nursing practice, could not adequately encompass nursing ethics. A nursing ethics needs to treat the call to care and how that call is inherent in nursing practice. In Chapter 4, we interpret that call philosophically in a way that does not require religious calling but does not exclude it.

In Chapter 5, we attempt to show that any adequate nursing ethics is therapeutic. A nursing ethics that takes seriously the moral sense of nursing will be a therapeutic ethics. Ethics is not usually considered to be therapeutic. Even Richard Zaner (1988), who designated his ethics a clinical ethics, seemed unaware of the therapeutic thrust of his ethics. When we interpreted his description of his work as an ethicist in clinical practice (Zaner 1993), we came to the conclusion that his ethics is a therapeutic one. This insight led us to interpret nursing ethics as a therapeutic ethics, which we attempt to demonstrate by interpretation of several examples.

Chapter 6 begins with a brief summary of the book. Then it shifts to a dialogue between the authors. The purpose of that dialogue, as well as that of this book, is to explore the possibility of an ethics that grows out of the moral dimension of nursing, one that helps practicing nurses recognize and realize the moral sense of practice. This dialogical approach allows the authors to speak from their own particular perspectives, rather than from the common perspective usually expressed as "we." Anne, one of the authors, speaks from the perspective of a practicing nurse with extensive experience in nursing education and a clinical specialty in psychiatric nursing. Jack, the other author, brings to their dialogue the perspective of a philosopher who, as a specialist in phenomenology of the human sciences, has written extensively on the philosophy of education. Although both are committed to feminist values, they speak from long experience of situations in which the separation of men and women and male dominance were taken for granted. For over fifteen years, they have been engaged in an ongoing dialogue concerning the meaning of nursing, in which each of the partners speaks out of his or her own particular experience. Since this dialogue is a personal one as well as one between a philosopher and a nurse, we have chosen to designate the participants personally as Jack and Anne. We will initiate this dialogical approach in the remainder of the chapter and then return to it in the final chapter.

Dialogical Interpretation

Jack: I think that the way you became involved in ethics is more interesting than my involvement in ethics. After all, ethics is one of the primary fields of interest of philosophers.

Anne: It is difficult to be a nurse and not consider moral
            issues. I know it is fashionable to say that interest in
            ethics came from advances in biomedical technol-
            ogy, but nursing as I have known it always involved
            moral concerns.

Jack: Advances in biomedical technology could not be the
            source of moral concerns in nursing if, as we claim,
            nursing has an inherent moral sense. However,
            advances in biomedical technology have certainly
            made health care workers more aware of the moral
            issues inherent in their practice.

Anne: When these issues became urgent, nurses turned to
            philosophers for help. I suppose that's why books
            on nursing ethics have tended to be applied ethics.

Jack: As I remember it, your first encounter with philo-
            sophical ethics took the applied approach.

Anne: Yes, I used one of the first texts that applied philo-
            sophical ethics to nursing ethics during a seminar
            designed to introduce nursing leaders to ethical
            thinking.

Jack: I remember when you returned from the seminar.
            You proudly asserted that now you were ready to
            argue with me about ethical issues in nursing.

Anne: Then you asked a crucial question: Did the work of
            the seminar prepare me to help nursing students
            recognize and resolve the issues they face in nursing
            practice? I responded, "No," but I think that you
            already knew that I would.

Jack: I remember all your frantic phone calls requesting
            help in understanding the meaning of Kantian
            autonomy and utilitarianism. It sounded like a
            typical course in ethics taught by a philosopher, and
            I remember wondering how it was specifically
            related to nursing practice. That's why I asked you
            whether it would help you introduce nursing
            students to ethical issues confronted in nursing
            practice.

Anne: In the seminar, we examined problems that were
            supposedly typical of the ethical problems that

nurses face in practice. Autonomy ethics and utilitarian ethics sometimes seemed to speak to some of these problems.

Jack: With all the stress on patients' rights, I can see why an autonomy ethics would speak to certain kinds of problems. These problems often deal with situations in which what the patient wants conflicts with what the nurse or physician thinks is best for the patient's health. Advocates of patients' rights draw on Kant because Kant insisted that every human being should be treated as an end, never merely as a means, and that making moral decisions required freedom to make the decisions.

Anne: The patients' rights movement assumes that all patients have the right to decide what will be done to them, even when it goes against the best health care practice.

Jack: Advocates of utilitarianism often find themselves in conflict with advocates of rights. The utilitarian believes that we should make decisions that foster the greatest good for the greatest number. Often this means denying the rights of a particular patient for the good of all.

Anne: Didn't you once refer me to an article in which an ethicist used autonomy ethics as well as utilitarian ethics to argue against allowing a patient to decide not to be treated?

Jack: That article came from a book that was specifically designed to demonstrate the contribution of applied philosophy to various types of human endeavors. In that example, Perry, a medical ethicist, is confronted with an unusual case. A patient who had been admitted to the hospital with a broken bone began to engage in bizarre behavior. An examination of his records showed a past history of mania that had been successfully treated with Lithium. When the patient was given Lithium, he became rationally competent to make decisions. In a rational state, he demanded that the Lithium treatment be stopped, because he enjoyed being in the manic state. An ethicist was called in to assess the moral issues involved in this case. The ethicist considered the case from the point of view of both utilitarianism and Kantian autonomy. After arguing that utilitarianism would favor treatment, he then considered Kantian ethics. First, he argued that a Kantian autonomy ethics favored non-treatment, since the patient, while in a rational state, decided he did not want to be treated. Then, the ethicist raised the issue of whether a person has the right to use autonomy to deny any possible future autonomy. If autonomy or self-direction is the highest good, can one legitimately use this claim to preclude future ability to make autonomous decisions? Ethicists often treat this problem as the issue of "does one have the right to sell oneself into slavery?" The ethicist in this case concluded that one does not have such a right, and therefore the patient should be treated.

Anne: Did the physicians follow the ethicist's recommendation?

Jack: No, they ignored both arguments.

Anne: I'm not surprised, since he completely failed to address the clinical situation. What decision did the physicians make?

Jack: They decided to treat the patient on the basis of third-party considerations, namely, that non-treatment would impose an undue burden on the family and health care facilities. In presenting this case as an example of applied ethics, the ethicist did not even raise the issue of why the physicians ignored his ingenious and well-developed arguments .

Anne: Wasn't he concerned about how the physicians arrived at their decision or about the adequacy of their decision?

Jack: No, he didn't discuss either. But it seems clear that the physicians as practitioners were primarily concerned with the well-being of the patient and those who must care for him, and not with ingenious philosophical arguments.

Anne: I think that the physicians were right in being concerned with the well-being of the patient and those who cared for him. Nursing needs an approach to ethics that speaks directly to practitioners and takes seriously the moral sense of nursing.

Jack: Does this mean that you think that the applied approach has little to offer nursing?

Anne: No, I think I benefited greatly from participating in a seminar on the applied approach. But, I do not believe that the applied approach should be the only approach. Moral decisions are required by the nature of nursing practice, and nurses are continually faced with decisions of moral import. My concern is that those who use the applied approach tend to neglect the process of nursing. For example, nursing is usually concerned with an ongoing process in which there is continual interaction between the patient and nurse, not with problems that can be solved in a once-and-for-all fashion.

Jack: It seems to me that what's often called a moral problem in nursing could more appropriately be called a moral dilemma. In nursing practice, aren't nurses more often confronted with moral situations and dilemmas than with moral problems?

Anne: Yes. Most issues in nursing ethics cannot be solved as problems, but must be responded to in ongoing situations. In these ongoing situations, there are possibilities for expanding and enhancing client well-being. In a problematic approach, nurses look for solutions rather than for possibilities that enhance and expand the practitioner's ability to foster patient well-being in an ongoing and developing process.

Jack: Most of the cases I have examined in nursing ethics books are chosen to illustrate types of philosophical thinking, rather than issues encountered in typical nursing practice.

Anne: Many cases chosen for ethical examination refer to a past situation. Nurses are concerned with present decisions, actions, and interpersonal relationships that are directed toward improving future health, not with what has happened in the past. And even when these cases are directed toward the future, they are treated as if a once-and-for-all decision is going to be made. For example, there is much talk in health care ethics about informed consent. The pattern for informed consent seems to come from granting permission to do medical or surgical procedures.

Jack: Do you mean that the patient signs a form that says to the physician, in effect, that it is okay to "do it to me"? Presumably, such consent assumes that I have been informed about what will be done to me and the risks involved.

Anne: The "do it to me" aspect of informed consent assumes that this is a once-and-for-all procedure, such as having your appendix removed. "Informing consent" makes more sense in nursing practice than informed consent. Nurses have to continually inform patients about what they are going to do to and with them, and continually need their tacit, if not explicit, consent. The purpose of informing consent is to foster cooperative relationships between patient and nurse, not merely to respect patient rights. Cooperative relationships are required for healing to take place, for pain to be relieved, or for hope to be restored.

Jack: Actually, informing consent might make more sense than informed consent in medical ethics. Regardless, the appropriateness of informing consent for nursing practice indicates why nursing ethics should take seriously the way in which nursing is practiced.

Anne: In fact, our concern with ethics has grown out of our attempt to make sense out of nursing as it is practiced. In both of our previous books, we have shown not only that nursing is a practice with an inherent moral sense, but that most nurses, at least implicitly, recognize that moral sense.

Jack: Most human endeavors have a dominant sense, which is only sometimes a moral one. In a free enterprise economy, the dominant sense of business is making profit for the owners. In business, ethics concerns matters that are adjunct to profit making, such as, how much a business can pollute the environment or endanger workers and clients in pursuing profit.

Anne: If in business, ethical issues are adjunct to profit making, those in business with strong moral commitments are in a tenuous situation.

Jack: Let me illustrate with an example. I attempted to purchase a used car to replace the old car with which I "limped" through graduate school. I asked a friend, who was in charge of sales for a car dealer, to find me a used car that I could afford. My friend took me to the used car lot and told me that he would not sell me any car on the lot, because I was his friend, but that he would find me a good affordable car. As we left the lot, my friend posed the question, "I have to sell all of those cars at a profit. The well-being of my family depends on it. You are supposed to know about ethics. Tell me, how can I do that and live by the Golden Rule?" My friend's dilemma resulted from being committed to an ethics that required him to help others, while being in an occupation that required him to make as much profit as possible for his employers. Unlike my friend, a nurse engages in a practice that is designed to foster the well-being of others. That's one meaning of nursing's having a dominant moral sense.

Anne: But that does not imply that nurses do not face moral tension in trying to fulfill the moral sense. A nursing scholar used this tension to challenge my assertion, in a paper I delivered, that nursing is a practice with a dominant moral sense. She stated, "Practicing nurses feel guilty when they view your philosophy of nursing as nursing's having a moral sense!" And then she asked, "What happens when nurses can't always practice morally?"

Jack: That is a strange response to our contention that nursing has a dominant moral sense.

Anne: Nurses feel guilty because they know that much of what they do has direct and indirect effects on patient well-being. When they fail to fulfill the moral sense, they feel guilty. This guilt is often dulled by routine procedures and technical and professional language that obscure the moral sense. Nurses feel less guilty when they can say, "I did this according to standard procedures," or "I did it using the latest technology," rather than saying, "I'm morally responsible for ensuring that my care fosters the well-being of my patient." The guilt that nurses feel, when they recognize the inadequacy of their care, results from being engaged in a practice that positively seeks to foster the well-being of others. Our stress on the moral sense makes nurses aware of their moral responsibility.

Jack: My friend, the used car salesman, would gladly face the guilt that nurses face. He would like nothing better than to be in a profession that calls for fostering the well-being of others, and hence matches his Christian morality. My friend would think it strange that nurses feel guilty when they discover the moral sense of nursing. Given his commitment to foster the well-being of others, my friend would find it fulfilling to be in a practice in which he could be an excellent practitioner and at the same time fulfill his moral commitment to the well-being of others.

Anne: An ethics for nursing should be different from a business ethics, but I feel that in some ways they are becoming similar.

Jack: Is that because of the emphasis on balancing the budget in hospitals and other health care institutions, and the fee system used in paying physicians and others?

Anne: Those are significant factors, but that's not primarily what I had in mind. Often I have the feeling that nurses and physicians talk and sometimes act as if they are engaged in a purely professional or technical activity, and that moral issues come up as side issues in the same way that they do in business.

Jack: That certainly matches the bioethics approach, in which ethical issues are generally regarded as coming about as a result of advances in modern technology. This, of course, implies that medicine, and perhaps nursing, is a technological activity that occasionally spawns moral problems requiring the help of experts called ethicists.

Anne: When nursing is regarded as a technological activity, then moral concerns become adjunct to that activity as they are in business. When the primary sense of an activity, such as nursing, is a moral sense, moral considerations are the primary concern and focus.

Jack: Since this is so, an ethics suitable to nursing should stress actual cases that disclose how the moral sense of nursing is fulfilled. In attempting to disclose the moral sense of nursing, we have interpreted many different examples of good nursing in our previous articles and books. This book is needed to expand that articulation of the moral sense of nursing by considering examples that show the ethical import of fulfilling the moral sense.

Anne: I don't see how we could adequately treat nursing ethics without interpreting examples of good nursing that disclose how the moral sense of nursing is fulfilled. Nurses make many moral decisions each day concerning practice. Examples from practice can disclose how the moral sense of practice can be fulfilled in ways that will encourage better practice.

Jack: Our stress on concrete examples should not imply that we neglect philosophical treatments of the meaning of being human. Philosophy can enhance our understanding of the meaning of nursing and nursing ethics. Our interpretation of nursing as a practice with an inherent moral sense drew heavily on Hans-Georg Gadamer's philosophy.

Anne: Also, our contention that nursing is the practice of caring drew on the feminist philosophies of caring of Carol Gilligan and Nel Noddings.

Jack: But we did not attempt to found nursing on these philosophies. Instead, they enlightened our understanding of the meaning of nursing as practiced. In this book, in addition to Gadamer, Gilligan and Noddings, Patricia Benner, Martin Buber, Richard Zaner, William James, Werner Marx, and Charles Taylor enhance our understanding of nursing ethics.

Anne: Noddings enlightened our understanding of nursing, by describing caring and relating it to ethics.

Jack: Gilligan supplied a context for our in-between stance, in which nurses work in-between physician, patient, and administrator. She shows why the in-between does not imply subservience to males. She argues that male thought is hierarchical and assumes that each person will strive to be alone at the top in order to be autonomous. In contrast, feminine values foster cooperation, interaction, and mutual support. Consequently, human beings should seek to be in-between, where they can support each other and foster cooperative interactions that promote each other's well-being.

Anne: Hierarchical systems based upon one highest value tend to distort nursing practice. In nursing as practiced, there are many values, some of which become more important than others in given contexts. For instance, a patient in excruciating pain wants more than anything else for the pain to end. A good nurse will usually do all that is possible to diminish the pain. That doesn't make the nurse or the patient a hedonist who contends that experiencing pleasure and avoiding pain are the highest good.

Jack: The fact that autonomy is of little concern to the patient who is enduring excruciating pain does not mean that autonomy is not to be highly prized in other circumstances.

Anne: Nurses value autonomy when physicians and hospital bureaucrats attempt to direct their nursing care. But some nurses seem to want autonomy because they think that being professional requires it, rather than because fostering the well-being of patients requires it.

Jack: I have often suspected that some nurses value the principle of autonomy as a means of supporting their conviction that the profession of nursing should have greater self-direction, rather than from philosophic commitment to that principle.

Anne: That suspicion probably came from the heat that was aroused in some nursing circles by the treatment of autonomy in our 1987 study.

Jack: I must admit that I found it confusing to be charged with being an enemy of autonomy.

Anne: Knowing how zealously you defend the right of self-direction, I can understand that. But being a woman in nursing, I understand why contemporary nurses stress autonomy and are suspicious of the in-between stance. Women, at least of my generation, were expected to serve those that we were in-between, with little self-direction. Physicians, and later hospital administrators, expected nurses to assume a subservient role. Now nurses are understandably demanding greater autonomy.

Jack: They deserve it! But we were not arguing against autonomy. We contended that nursing as a caring practice intends the physical and psychological well-being of others, and that greater autonomy is needed to fulfill the moral sense of nursing. Thus autonomy, although necessary to fulfill the moral sense, cannot constitute the primary sense of nursing or nursing ethics.

Anne: Nurses do need greater professional autonomy in order to bring about needed reform in patient care. Reformers are understandably suspicious of a philosophy of nursing that reaffirms traditional nursing values. I can understand why our stress on deriving the meaning of nursing from actual practice has led many nurses to label us as traditionalists. Nurses have struggled hard and long against a tradition that confined them, as nurses and as women, to a subservient way of being. They tend to hear valuing tradition as "traditional," even when the return to the past is a source of reform.

Jack: Most of the major reform movements, at least in the Western world, have come from seeing new possibilities in traditional values that have been neglected or distorted by changing times.

Anne: We nurses are recovering the centrality of caring in the nursing tradition that has been lost due to the stress on science, technology, and bureaucracy.

Jack: The stress on instrumental reasoning in technology and bureaucracy can obscure the moral sense, but caring discloses it.

Anne: The recovery of nursing as essentially caring is directing us to the moral sense of nursing as it is encountered in practice and shared with colleagues.

Jack: To hear some health care ethicists, you would think that advances in technology and bureaucracy created the need for ethics.

Anne: But they have the cart before the horse. Health care grew out of the need to care for the ill and debilitated in a given time and situation. In our time and situation, technological advance and administrative efficiency have become necessary for adequate health care. Although they have contributed much to the fulfillment of the moral sense of health care, they have, at the same time, tended to obscure its importance.

Jack: When people talk about advances in health care, they almost always speak of scientific and technological improvement. Why do we omit contributions that have come from humanistic understanding of persons?

Anne: It seems to me that nursing has been much improved by the stress on open disclosure, developing personal relationships, cooperative interactions, and authenticity.

Jack: Patients and their families have certainly benefited from such understanding. I remember when visiting a hospital was somewhat like entering an army post.

You needed a pass to get in, and children were forbidden. Now hospitals are much more open.

Anne: Gaining information about treatment was almost impossible except when it was given by a physician in brief conferences full of technical language. Nurses never told patients what medications they were on or what their blood pressure was. The only response the nurse could give was, "You'll have to talk to your doctor." Now, with the increased openness, nurses are able to share understanding with patients as human beings do in normal conversation.

Jack: Humanistic understanding has led to the recovery of the moral sense of nursing. Keeping the moral sense of health care focal is one of the most important contributions that ethics can make to health care.

Anne: I want that contribution to be focused on nursing as well as on ethics. When ethics concerns nursing, I want moral decisions, actions, and relationships to be considered as I encounter them in clinical situations.

Jack: When I do ethics, I want to consider something that's going on in the world that should foster the well-being of persons. When I teach ethics, I like to be philosophically engaged in exploring the meaning of the good as it is encountered in the world, rather than as it has been distilled from the works of the great philosophers. My favorite ethics class was one in which our professor developed his own ethics and required us to explore and criticize the great classical ethical philosophies on our own. My only regret was that he did not give his ethics in written form so that it could be digested before class sessions, and its adequacy and possibilities be discussed in an ongoing dialogue in class.

Anne: When our book is used as a text, should it be used in the way you wish your professor had chosen? What difference does it make that those who use our book will not be its authors?

Jack: The issue, for me, is not who authored the text. I have used texts written by ethics professors that

rehashed what past ethicists have said, criticized
their ethics, and made suggestions for practical
applications. Rather than taking that approach, my
favorite professor invited us to think with him about
the meaning of being moral.

Anne: Our book is primarily an original interpretation of
nursing ethics that begins with the moral sense of
nursing. It is primarily directed towards the world
rather than the classroom. Isn't it difficult for such a
book to be a textbook? Didn't you and Al Mickunas
run into a problem in trying to write a book that was
a philosophical interpretation of education and at
the same time a text?

Jack: We sure did. Our editor demanded that we decide
whether the book was a text or a contribution to
knowledge. Since the book was about 80% contribution to knowledge and 20% text, it was not difficult
for us to make the choice and eliminate the text-like
chapter from the book. Seriously, that book, like this
one, was not originally written as either a textbook
or a contribution to knowledge, although those who
think in these terms would probably call it a contribution to knowledge.

Anne: I never thought of contributing to knowledge when
we proposed this book. We wrote the book to
explore the possibility of an ethics that grows out of
and focuses on the moral sense of nursing. Such
original explorations are usually aimed at specialists
in colleges and universities, and are written in their
customary language. We are attempting to avoid
technical language and academic "insider" knowledge in order to speak to practicing nurses and
students as well as scholars. Consequently, one
answer to the question posed by the title of this
chapter, "Why Another Book on Nursing Ethics?" is
that this book is different from other books on ethics
in that it is an original investigation of nursing ethics
that seeks to involve students and nurses in that
exploration.

Jack: I hope that through sharing in our explorations,
practicing nurses and students will recognize and

realize the moral sense of their practice in ways that will enhance their abilities to engage in ethical considerations. By ethical considerations, I mean the ability to lift out the moral significance of their practice and to develop facility in understanding how to fulfill the moral imperatives in their practice. I also hope that students of ethics will learn to take seriously the moral sense embedded in practices.

Anne: I applaud the stress on understanding the ethical dimensions of practice, but I want more than understanding of the moral sense and its implications for practice. I hope that our articulation of nursing ethics will call nurses to thoughtful care for patients and for the practice of nursing. I especially want nurses to care thoughtfully for the moral sense of practice that seems to be waning in this time of stress on technology and professionalism.

Study Hints

1. Read the first and sixth chapters as though you were part of this dialogue with Jack and Anne. As you read the dialogue, questions or comments will come to your mind. Write them for consideration in in-class discussion.
2. Read each chapter and then read the portion of Chapter 6 that discusses the major cases presented in the chapter, in order to consider them in a broader ethical context.

Study Questions

1. What are the major themes that Anne and Jack will develop in this book?
2. Why does Anne think that a traditional ethics focused on past cases is inadequate for making ethical judgments concerning nursing practice?
3. Why does Anne believe that informing consent is more appropriate for nursing practice than informed consent?
4. Why would the used car salesman who is committed to the Golden Rule find it strange that nurses feel guilty because nursing has a moral sense?

5. Why do some nurses feel guilty when reminded that nursing has a moral sense? Do you agree with them? Why or why not?
6. Why does Anne believe that ethics in nursing is sometimes treated as it is in business?
7. What inadequacies in applied ethics are evident in the case of the ethicist who developed an ingenious argument from the principle of autonomy for treatment for the patient with mania?
8. Why do Jack and Anne believe that most moral problems in nursing ethics are more appropriately called moral dilemmas?
9. What do Anne and Jack mean by practice? Do you believe that nursing is a practice? Why or why not?
10. What reasons do Anne and Jack give for writing this book? What are some other reasons for writing a book on nursing ethics?
11. What is meant by the in-between stance of nursing, and what contribution does Gilligan's philosophy make to it?
12. Why does Anne believe that contemporary nurses stress autonomy and distrust traditional and in-between stances?
13. Why do Anne and Jack favor the use of examples to disclose the meaning of being a good nurse?
14. Why has the recovery of caring led to a recovery of the moral sense of nursing?
15. What do Jack and Anne mean by their contention that humanistic understanding has led to the improvement of health care? Do you agree with their contention? Why or why not?
16. How do Jack and Anne believe this book differs from traditional ethics textbooks?
17. What do Anne and Jack hope will result from study of their book?

References

Bishop, Anne H., and John R. Scudder, Jr. (1990). *The Practical, Moral, and Personal Sense of Nursing: A Phenomenological Philosophy of Practice*. Albany, N.Y. : State University of New York Press.

Bishop, Anne H., and John R. Scudder, Jr. (1991). *Nursing: The Practice of Caring*. New York: The National League for Nursing Press.

Gadamer, Hans-Georg. (1981). *Reason in the Age of Science* . trans. F. G. Lawrence. Cambridge, Mass.: MIT Press.

Gilligan, Carol. (1982). *In a Different Voice: Psychological Theory and Women's Development*. Cambridge, Mass.: Harvard University Press.

Noddings, Nel. (1984). *Caring: A Feminine Approach to Ethics and Moral Education*. Berkeley: University of California Press.

Perry, Clifton B. (1989). *The Philosopher as Medical Ethicist: Applying Ethical Theories.* In Philosophers at Work: An Introduction to the Issues and Practical Uses of Philosophy, ed. E.D. Cohen, 35–42. New York: Holt, Rinehart and Winston.

Zaner, Richard M. (1993). *Troubled Voices: Stories of Ethics and Illness.* Cleveland, Ohio: Pilgrim Press.

2

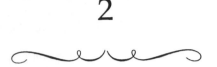

On Being a Good Nurse

The waning of the moral sense in nursing is evident in the meaning often attributed to statements concerning being a good nurse. "Good" used in this way rarely means being morally good but being attentive, effective, and efficient in the practice of nursing. If it refers to being morally good at all, good means well-motivated, in the sense of being concerned about the well-being of the patient.

A crucial moral issue in nursing ethics concerns the relationship of (1) "good" in the sense of attentive, efficient, and effective with (2) "good" in the personal sense. Good in the first sense usually means understanding the ways of the practice of nursing and employing them to foster the well-being of patients. Good in the second sense usually means that nursing care grows out of personal concern for the well-being of patients. Good in the first sense becomes synonymous with good in the second sense when nursing is interpreted as a caring practice. A practice consists of historically developed ways of fostering good in which the good sought, the ways of fostering that good, and the personal concern for the other are integrally related to each other. Thus, to say that a nurse is morally good means that she/he is actively concerned with fostering the patient's well-being through a caring relationship that requires attentive, efficient, and effective nursing practice.

Integral Nature of Nursing Practice

Unfortunately, the personal aspect of nursing is often separated from the practical aspect and is regarded as the true meaning of the moral sense. This bifurcation was assumed by the nursing scholar mentioned in Chapter 1, who stated that nurses feel guilty when we stress the moral sense of nursing. Nurses often feel guilty because they do not always feel compassion for patients for whom they care. This separation of the personal side of nursing from the impersonal—the technological and professional—is unsound and detrimental to nursing practice. It reduces morality to personal relationships divorced from the empowerment of nursing practice. A morally good nurse would certainly cultivate the methods and skills necessary to empower effective care. In excellent practice, good nurses do not separate empowerment from personal relations. They show their personal concern for patients by supporting and empowering them so that they can recover from illness, overcome debilitation, and live more healthfully. When nurses engage in excellent practice, they are caring for the well-being of persons. Conversely, they care for persons by engaging in excellent practice.

When care for persons is separated from practice, then a nurse is apt to say something like, "I care for the patient (I have a beneficent feeling toward the patient and therefore am a good moral being), and therefore I must develop a nursing care plan (I will be effective and efficient and therefore a good nurse)." Nursing care does not happen in this way. When a nurse sees the patient in pain, he/she does not say, "I have a feeling of concern for this patient's well-being, therefore I must give the pain medication." He/she responds immediately to the pain with the prescribed remedy. If asked why the patient is being treated that way, the nurse would merely explain that the patient is in pain, rather than saying, "I have a beneficent feeling for the patient." The good of the patient is built into the remedy, and the nurse knows that it is. The ways of the practice have the good of the patient built into them; hence, they have an inherent moral sense. When they are employed, care for the person is present from the beginning. Of course, nurses are not always overtly conscious of this presence, but it is tacitly present in their actions

In authentic nursing, good intentions are not separated from empowerment. When a nurse initially states, "I must do something to help this person," the empowering ability to do something is already present in her/his statement of commitment, although she/he may not be overtly conscious of it at the moment. What that empowering ability consists of depends upon the nurse and the situation.

When concern for well-being is separated from empowerment, then the moral good is usually limited to personal relationships from which empowering technical and professional competence are excluded. According to this way of thinking, the nurse is being moral when she/he cares for a patient personally, but not when he/she is efficiently using technology to foster the well-being of the patient. Nurses perform all kinds of activities efficiently and effectively that are not overtly connected to personal relationships or beneficent feelings. Nurses could hardly do otherwise. However, the well-being of the other is tacitly present in the activities and relationships that constitute nursing practice. Activities and relationships are moral in nursing when they are being done for the well-being of the other.

Many nurses see a clear relationship between morality and practice when they are personally attending to patients with the direct hands-on care that previously constituted much of nursing. But when engaged in complicated technological care, they find it difficult to recognize or feel the moral sense in that care. This is especially true in technical activities that require giving more attention to technique than to the patient. But nurses who work within the moral sense of practice recognize that temporarily focusing their attention away from the patient, to perform exacting procedures, is done for the good of the patient. It is not the nature of the activity—direct care or technical care—that makes it moral, but its being done for the well-being of the patient.

Since the moral sense is inherent in practice, it is possible for a nurse to contribute to fulfilling the moral sense of nursing without being moral herself/himself. For example, consider a nurse who has "gotten by" with a focus on the practical aspects of nursing with limited understanding of even the meaning of his/her work, much less of the meaning of nursing in a wider social context. Suppose also that the nurse works in a situation in which almost all of his/her work is prescribed by others, and that the nurse is primarily motivated by a desire to please superiors so that he/she can keep his/her job and possibly be promoted in it. In this case, the nurse would have no intentional involvement in fulfilling the moral sense of nursing. This would not mean that the nursing engaged in would have no moral sense, but instead that the nurse would not be a moral being when engaged in this moral practice. Such a nurse probably would consider herself/himself a moral being only when engaged in personal relations with patients outside of effective, efficient, and attentive practice.

An Outstanding Nurse

The relationship of being a good nurse in the moral sense to being a good nurse in the practical sense is evident in one of Benner's examples of nursing excellence. She uses this example to illustrate excellent nursing in the domain of Effective Management of Rapidly Changing Situations. [The other domains are The Helping Role, The Teaching-Coaching Function, The Diagnostic and Patient-Monitoring Function, Administering and Monitoring Therapeutic Interventions and Regimens, Monitoring and Ensuring the Quality of Health Care Practice, and Organizational and Work-Role Competencies (Benner 1984, 46).]

I came on duty at 3 PM and was assigned to a fresh postop open heart surgery. The patient had returned to the ICU around 11

AM that day and had all the usual paraphernalia for postops—IVs, respirator, chest tubes, foley catheters, etc. The patient had had a log [sic] of IV fluid and blood replacement on days—this is the usual procedure for open heart surgery—give lots of fluid at first (usually have had mannitol), then level off. Blood pressure will drop as the patient begins to warm up and dilate peripherally, but will usually level off soon. However, this patient continued to be hypovolemic—low blood pressure, low central venous pressure—and was diuresing in enormous amounts. We were pouring fluids in, in an attempt to catch up, but were managing, barely, to stay even with output. The patient by this time (4:30–5 PM) was fully warm, so clearly something else was amiss here. I telephoned the surgeon's exchange but was not able to locate him. The exchange promised that they would have him call as soon as possible. I tried also to contact the assistant, but he was off call to another doctor who was not terribly familiar with open heart surgery. Meanwhile, we were pouring in fluids, blood and packed cells, without orders, just to stay even, for the patient was continuing this diuresis. I began reviewing the possible causes for this and decided a likely one was hyperglycemia. I then ordered a blood glucose level and the results came back—more than 600 mg percent. About this time the assistant surgeon had come back on call and I was finally able to contact him. He prescribed for the patient on the basis of the blood glucose level and we were then able to stabilize the patient. (Benner 1984, 116–117)

From *From Novice to Expert* by Patricia Benner. Copyright (©) 1984 by Addison-Wesley Publishing Company. Reprinted by permission.

This is certainly an example of effective nursing, but it is also an example of morally good nursing. The nurse's decisions and actions are directed at fostering the well-being of the patient. She gives the direction, without orders, necessary to keep her patient alive. When she is unable to secure a physician, she makes her own diagnosis and acts by ordering a blood glucose level. But why does this make her a morally good person? She has not used the Kantian or utilitarian norms to make her judgment; in fact, these norms seem irrelevant to the many decisions she makes in response to changing conditions. She is a morally good person because she effectively decides and acts to foster the well-being of the patient. The goodness of her acts stands out, and is therefore outstanding, because she takes risks by proceeding without orders when they are unavailable but needed to foster the well-being of the patient. Are only such outstanding decisions and acts moral care? Certainly not! Nurses continually, by diligent and effective care, foster the well-being of patients. Most nursing consists of just such care. But outstanding care makes the moral sense that is inherent in ordinary care stand out. Nurses are daily called on to routinely foster the well-being of patients. Only occasionally is that commitment tested by an unusual situation. The nurse in the above case could have failed the test by playing it safe. She could have reasoned that nurses should not act without medical orders, much less make diagnoses and issue orders. She probably would contend that a morally good nurse gives extra personal attention to patients. Consequently, she would hold the patient's hand, mop his brow, and pray for his well-being. However, her playing it safe would disclose that her primary concern is not for the well-being of the patient but for legalistically "doing what nurses are supposed to do." Her decisions and actions would disclose *her* meaning of a good nurse. For her, a good nurse stays safely within limits set by others and gives extra personal attention to the patient. She does not, as the nurse in the above example did, take risks to foster the well-being of patients. It is not taking risks that makes a nurse morally good, but the devotion to fostering the well-being of the patient that requires taking risks when the situation calls for it.

The Moral Sense of Competency

Fulfillment of the moral sense of nursing occurs in competent care as well as in outstanding care. Much of the fostering of the well-being of patients by nurses occurs in competent care. When the tacit presence of "for the well-being of others" is obscured by work that has become routine, or by a context of professional and technical non-moral systems of meaning, work becomes boring and burnout often occurs. An example of this is evident in the following description of a nurse's most fulfilling experience.

The most fulfilling experience I ever had was when a child I was caring for arrested but was successfully resuscitated. I had written my notice that day—I wanted out of nursing—it was killing me. The baby stopped breathing while we were on the elevator coming back from X-ray. I did mouth-to-mouth on her until we got back to the room and the code team arrived. The baby responded beautifully. Naturally I felt good. But when the mother praised me for "saving" her baby, I tried to tell her that what I did was not so special; anyone can do mouth-to-mouth.

"But it was you," she said. "You were there. If you hadn't wanted to be a nurse in the first place and been working that day, I wouldn't have my baby." (Bishop and Scudder 1990, 101)

Excerpted from *The Practical, Moral, and Personal Sense of Nursing* by Bishop, A. H. and Scudder, J. R., Jr. © 1990 State University of New York. Reprinted by permission of SUNY Press.

The nurse in the above example decided to return to nursing when she recognized the moral sense inherent in competent nursing practice. Those who think that the tensions that cause burnout come from caring will find the above example strange. This would not seem strange to Benner and Wrubel since they contend that it "is a peculiarly modern mistake to think that caring is the cause of burnout." They contend that, as the above story discloses, "the return of caring is the recovery" from burnout (Benner and Wrubel 1989, 373).

It is significant that, in the above example, the nurse's recovery from burnout occurred when she recognized the moral sense in competent care rather than in excellent care. As the nurse said, "Anyone [presumably meaning any competent nurse] can do mouth-to-mouth." The mother's gratitude for the saving of her child led the nurse to recognize the moral sense inherent even in routine nursing practice. When this happened, the nurse recognized that the good in competent practice and the moral good were one and the same, and she decided to remain in nursing.

From Competency to Excellence

The first moral obligation of a nurse is to become a competent practitioner. Incompetent nurses do harm. One of the ancient maxims in health care is "to do no harm." Competency refers to the minimum requirements for being a nurse. Nursing students and novice practitioners have as their primary obligation to reach the level of competency.

When nurses reach the level of competency, they are tempted to remain there rather than face the risks of authentic care. As Benner and Wrubel point out, "the risk and vulnerability inherent in caring lead to the temptation to create safe places of 'controlled caring'" (Benner and Wrubel 1989, 2). One of the safest places for a veteran nurse to control care is at the level of competent care. Then care becomes routine and loses the connection with concern that is present in novice nursing care. Competent practicing nurses have as their moral obligation to become excellent practitioners. Being a good nurse implies moving beyond competency toward becoming an excellent practitioner.

Since being a morally good nurse depends on the relationship between experience and attainment, becoming a good nurse should be interpreted in light of a nurse's movement from novice to expert. Benner (1984) has described this movement in nursing, drawing on the work of Hubert Dreyfus and Stuart Dreyfus. Dreyfus and Dreyfus (1991) have shown that morality itself presupposes such a development. In moving from a novice to an expert in ethics, persons first learn to follow the rules that commonly are regarded as the ethics of the community. Then, they act by following community maxims in the context of the situations in which they are involved. Finally, at the highest stage, rather than following the dictates of rules and principles, they make intuitive judgments concerning the right actions to take when encountering moral dilemmas and situations (Dreyfus and Dreyfus 1991, 236–237). Making intuitive judgments is recognizing the right thing to do without overtly going through all the rational processes involved in applying principles to practice.

Rather than following the traditional view that morally mature persons apply detached rational principles to moral problems, Dreyfus and Dreyfus contend that a morally mature person intuitively knows what to do, drawing on past experience. They also point out that a contextual intuitive ethics is the ethics of everyday moral life. This approach speaks directly to our attempt to develop an ethics that is appropriate to nurses in everyday practice.

This does not mean that learning to make moral judgments on the basis of principles is unimportant to the moral life. Novice nurses do need to learn how to make moral judgments, how to justify them rationally, and how to incorporate these abilities within their moral experience. Principled approaches to ethics teach nurses to value justice, rights, and autonomy, and to recognize situations in which justice, rights, and autonomy are involved, even when it is no longer necessary to follow them as principles to direct moral behavior. In clinical situations, nurses need to make intuitive decisions that draw on their past experience in order to foster the well-being of their clients. This moral experience needs to include the traditional moral wisdom of the community and ethical sensibilities developed during active participation in the moral life of that community.

The need to draw on general principles and common moral wisdom in making moral decisions should not keep nurses from consideration of the uniqueness of individuals and their situations, according to Dreyfus and Dreyfus.

> Each person must simply respond as well as he or she can to each unique situation with nothing but experience-based intuition as guide. Heidegger

... captures this ethical skill in his notion of *authentic care* as a response to
the *unique*, as opposed to the *general*, situation. Authentic caring in this
sense is common to *agape* and *phronesis*. (Dreyfus and Dreyfus 1991, 246)

Caring that is activated by *agape* and informed by *phronesis* is well-suited for
a nursing ethics. *Agape* is a passionate concern for the well-being of others,
and *phronesis* is practical wisdom that enables one to foster the other's well-
being.

Practical Wisdom

Since, in this chapter, we are attempting to show that the know-how of
nursing practice and that of nursing ethics are integrally related, we will
focus on what philosophers have traditionally called practical wisdom. To
identify a human activity as a practice, according to Gadamer (1981), means
that it is designed to foster human good. In that fostering of human good,
the ends sought and the way of achieving the good are one and the same.
The Greeks used the word "phronesis" to name the know-how that fosters
the good (Gadamer 1981).

Making moral decisions and practical decisions in nursing both require
intuitive judgment that draws on experience. Benner (1984) has shown that
making intuitive decisions by drawing on experience is characteristic of
excellent nursing. Dreyfus and Dreyfus have shown that a similar process
is involved in making moral decisions. In a practice in which the practical
and moral senses are so integrally related that making decisions about one
is making a decision about the other, it is helpful to employ the same way
of making judgments. The consequence of trying to make moral and
practical decisions in different ways was evident in the example in Chapter
1 that involved the issue of whether the patient with mania should be forced
to take Lithium. In making a decision to prescribe Lithium for the patient
with mania, the physicians ignored the ethicist's ingenious ethical argument
regarding autonomy. This argument, derived from rationalist philosophy,
seemed an irrelevant intrusion into clinical practice to the physicians who
were engrossed in making practical decisions that their previous experience
indicated would foster the good of all concerned.

Acting "As If"

The ethicist in the above case was using philosophical argument to arrive at
the answer deduced from the principle of autonomy, whereas the physicians were merely attempting to find the best answer given the clinical

situation. Most clinical situations involve change and uncertainty rather than static known situations, as Marianne Paget (1988) has pointed out in her exploration of errors in judgment by physicians. Unfortunately, much of traditional ethics assumes fixed known situations. Usually these situations are made static by dealing with past events or fixed hypothetical situations. When nurses and nursing students examine these static cases, they inevitably want more information than is provided in the description of the situation. They don't want to stay within the parameters set by the case. They tend to seek more satisfactory resolutions than provided by the alternatives set in the case. They ask, "What if it happened this way?" "What if someone felt this way?" or "What if someone did it this way?" This way of reasoning comes from dealing with concrete situations in which change is still possible and the future is to some degree unknown. In practice, nurses make decisions directed at an unknown future.

Paget has shown that health care involves acting in time. She contended that most medical prescriptions are given on an "as if" basis. Physicians proceed with treatment "as if" these treatments will benefit the patient, but they do not know in advance that they will. Nurses are well aware of the need to act "as if" without knowing the results in advance. This is evident in the following case of a nurse who let her physician-patient sleep rather than awakening him for chest physical therapy, because her experience in similar situations indicated that sleep was often more beneficial than physical therapy.

I took care of a patient, a very likable young physician, who had an open-and-close exploratory laparotomy for pancreatic cancer. He had been febrile. For three nights I woke him every four hours and helped him do all his breathing exercises and lung physical therapy. He was really depressed and wasn't talking about anything that had to do with his diagnosis and everything that was happening to him. The fourth night that I was on, his temperature had come down some, and by now he was exhausted from lack of sleep. I figured that he was going to have a lot better chance to focus on things that he needed and wanted to focus on if he could just get some uninterrupted sleep. His temperature remained the same in the morning. His lungs probably would have been clearer had I awakened him at 3 AM but I elected not to, given his extreme fatigue and depression. It's not clear what is the right thing to do. There are little studies done about the effectiveness of chest physical therapy and then there are other studies done about the effectiveness of sleep. But there is never anything that proves that X is better than Y, especially in a particular situation, so that I know that chest physical therapy every four hours is really going to help or that sleep is going to help. It is expected that I will use my best judgment under the circumstances. (Benner 1984, 140–141)

From *From Novice to Expert* by Patricia Benner. Copyright © 1984 by Addison-Wesley Publishing Company. Reprinted by permission.

In the above case, it is almost impossible to separate the moral from the practical. The nurse in this case is drawing on her past experience in making judgments concerning patient care, judgments that are at once practical and moral. This case is focused on how best to treat *this* particular patient in *this* concrete situation. In deciding what to do about this patient's sleep, the nurse is not only concerned with his physical well-being but also with his ability to make decisions about his future care. Just as there is no X or Y judgment demonstrating which decision is therapeutically best, there are no ways of making moral judgments that will clearly indicate which is the morally right course to follow in this case. Perhaps the best indication of the nurse's high moral character is her willingness to make a judgment unsupported by rational props, when her long experience indicates that sleep is probably best for this particular person. Her outstanding care discloses the moral obligation to act "as if" nursing care will foster the well-being of the patient when thoughtful reflection indicates that it will, even though positive assurance is lacking.

Acting "as if," according to Paget, involves producing an effect in the world by "altering biological phenomena, limiting disability, restoring function, relieving pain, controlling a disease process, or stopping plague" (Paget 1988, 49). These treatments all intend a therapeutic effect that is shown to be "accurate or plausible or revealing" (52) when tested in clinical situations. Acting "as if" involves risks for the physician and the patient. The physician's interpretation is at risk since the consequence of treatment is unknown. In following the treatment, the patient risks loss of well-being and possibly life. Since "clinical" action forges into an unknown "future," its time structure is different from "the more exact science of hindsight" (Paget 1988, 56).

Much instruction in nursing ethics is conducted from the perspective of hindsight into an unchanging situation. But nurses in a clinical setting are faced with situations that involve "as if" judgments concerning future outcomes that they can rarely predict with certainty. Making such judgments is often inappropriately called *"clinical judgment*, a [medical] term that transforms action into a cognition" (Paget 1988, 53). When this occurs, the nurse focuses on reasoning to a single decision that will direct all future care. But such decision "is not a decision but a sequence of *acts of deciding* being described as though it were a single decision" (53). The term, clinical judgment, masks the fact that care involves reassessment of changing situations that require new decisions involving interactions between nurse and patient, nurse and physician, nurse and administration.

In-Between Stance of Nurses

Nurses, more than other health care workers, are aware of the need for cooperative interaction and are better prepared to foster it, because they often work in an in-between stance. We have described the in-between as day-to-day care through which nurses foster the patient's well-being by bringing together (1) the physician's plan of medical care, (2) the institution's policies and resources, and (3) the patient's view of the good life (Bishop and Scudder 1990). We also have contended that the in-between stance of nursing needs to be coupled with Patricia Benner's description of nursing as the pursuit of excellence inherent in nursing practice, in which nurses should have relative autonomy to direct their own practice (Benner 1984).

The in-between stance has been criticized by some nursing scholars as a regression of nursing to the handmaiden status of nurses as servants to physicians. They are especially troubled when the in-between stance is put in the context of our contention that the essence of nursing is the moral sense of fostering the well-being of others. The commitment of nurses to the well-being of others has made them subject to abuse. Requiring nurses to work in-between physicians, agency administration, and patients increases the possibility of repression. For example, all nurses have encountered physicians who believe that having the right to give medical orders gives them the right to order the nurse's time in other ways. Nurses are further subject to abuse by being thought of as women, who, in our society, have been traditionally habituated to serve others and to work cooperatively in that serving. Feminists' concerns and nursing's demands for greater autonomy have converged to question our contention that the in-between stance is needed to fulfill the moral sense of nursing.

Surprisingly, the strongest support for our contention that the in-between stance enhances, rather than limits, the fulfillment of the moral sense of nursing comes from the feminist philosophy of Gilligan (1982). Gilligan contends that traditional ethics has had a masculine hierarchical order rather than a feminine web of connection. In a hierarchical structure, the person who is alone at the top has the greatest autonomy. It follows that autonomy decreases as one moves away from the top of the hierarchy. But

Gilligan contends that women tend to value relationships and interaction rather than autonomous action and power. In Western philosophy, ethics has stressed autonomous decision making and individual action rather than relationships, interaction and cooperation. Thus, those who stress the need for autonomy in order to make moral decisions are following in the Western male philosophical tradition.

According to the autonomy principle of traditional ethics, nurses would lack power when they operate from an in-between stance. Consequently, those who stress autonomy often believe that it is desirable that nurses rid themselves of the in-between position. But fostering the well-being of patients often requires nurses to work from an in-between stance (for a more extensive treatment of this theme, see Bishop and Scudder 1990, 1991). In giving everyday care, nurses have to facilitate the medical orders of physicians, utilize the facilities within the policies and procedures established by the institution or agency, and recognize the patient's wishes for a good life. This in-between stance is a negative one for nurses only if they accept the hierarchical view. In terms of the interactive web of connection advocated by Gilligan, it is a highly valued position.

The in-between position is a privileged one from which to foster cooperative moral decisions by all involved. Difficult moral decisions should be made by teams involving the physician, nurse, patient, other professionals, representatives of the hospital and family, and, when available, an ethicist. Nurses are well situated to facilitate cooperative decision making, because they understand the medical position, the hospital's vested interest and facilities, and usually the patient's and family's desires. Furthermore, a nurse is accustomed to making in-between decisions that involve taking all of these various aspects into account. The nurse, as an authority in nursing care, has his/her particular contributions and legitimate authority to contribute to this decision. But when nurses make their primary stance gaining autonomy, they make sure that their position is heard and recognized above all others. Such assertions, although required at times, foster power struggles rather than cooperative decision making. Nurses are uniquely situated to prevent power struggles. They have had to learn how to think from the other's position in order to work with physicians, hospital administration, patients, and families in planning everyday care. They have had to work within what Gilligan calls "the web of connection" (Gilligan 1982, 62). This experience uniquely prepares them to help other health care professionals recognize that it is necessary to work within a web of connection to fulfill the moral sense of health care. Such recognition will not come from militant demands for autonomy, but from helping others see that fostering the well-being of patients requires cooperative decision making and action within a web of connection.

Unfortunately, most cases in ethics books involving cooperative decision making that deals with health care problems are focused on making once-and-for-all judgments such as when to "pull the plug." In actual health care practice, moral judgments can rarely be made on a once-and-for-all basis. This is especially true for nurses since they work in-between and constantly adjust their care according to patient situations. Often they have to adjust their care because it is given in relationship to medical prescription, institutional requirements, and patient and family desires. Occasionally it becomes necessary for nurses to challenge the prescriptions, requirements, and desires of other team members, while attempting to maintain the cooperative relationships necessary for patient care.

Margie Smith is a Good Nurse

A story by Margie Smith (1993) shows how nurses can foster needed cooperation while doggedly opposing questionable decisions made by others on the health care team. This story also provides a concrete summary of the major themes of this chapter.

Debra Cooper, 78 years old, was admitted to the geriatric rehabilitation unit with a left above-the-knee amputation which, like her previous right below-the-knee amputation (with a prosthesis), resulted from gangrene caused by type I diabetes. She also had congestive heart failure and some disorientation as a result of organic dementia. Margie Smith was Mrs. Cooper's primary nurse.

"Before her left amputation, Mrs. Cooper was able to take care of herself and even help her daughter, who lived with her, with housekeeping, care of the 'grandbabies,' as she liked to refer to them, and cooking. Despite her disorientation, Mrs. Cooper knew she was in the hospital and that our job, in her words, was to 'get me walking with my grandbabies again.'"

Motivated patient

"After working with Mrs. Cooper for a few days I was impressed by her. She was one of the most motivated and cooperative patients I've ever known. Sure, she sometimes thought it was 1943, but she'd learned how to get in and out of her wheelchair without having any legs, and could use the bedpan. She never stopped talking about her goal of walking with two artificial legs.

"As I worked with her, I noticed that Mrs. Cooper's right prosthesis appeared loose. Her stump would twist within the prosthesis during transfers from the bed or wheelchair. It was loose enough that there were times when she would be standing almost literally on the ankle of her prosthesis as it tilted away from her stump. When I asked her about this, she admitted that the prosthesis 'just didn't feel right.'"

When the occupational therapists confirmed Margie's observations regarding the prosthesis fit, she conferred with the physical therapist and physician, who disagreed and said that nothing could be done. Margie was completely surprised when a discharge order was written for Mrs. Cooper after only one week, with no team meeting to discuss her progress.

"There hadn't been any attempt made to consult the prosthetist about Mrs. Cooper's ill-fitting right prosthesis or to fit her with a left prosthesis. There wasn't enough time to finalize the necessary discharge teaching with her daughter. More important, there was no wheelchair available for Mrs. Cooper and no time to teach this formerly ambulatory patient how to use it. Personally, I had difficulty turning this once-independent, ambulatory, motivated, cooperative woman, who was making good progress, into a wheelchair bound patient after only one week—especially on the basis of the physician's opinion alone. This wasn't the reason I went into nursing. This wasn't the standard of care I needed to give.

"I talked about this with Mrs. Cooper's physician. His opinion was that Mrs. Cooper wasn't a good prosthesis candidate because of her disorientation. In response, I offered documented examples from all the nursing staff of Mrs. Cooper's ability to learn new skills and her extraordinary motivation to be independent. I also expressed concern over the fit of the right prosthesis and asked if the prosthetist had been consulted."

Despite his contention that Mrs. Cooper wasn't a good prosthesis candidate, the physician canceled the discharge order when Margie related that several members of the rehabilitation team had similar goals for Mrs. Cooper, including prosthetic and ambulation goals.

Margie and the occupational therapist continued to document major problems with the right prosthesis, while the physical therapist replaced Mrs. Cooper's stump socks with thicker ones every day or two. Although Margie requested a stump compression sock to begin preparing Mrs. Cooper for a left prosthesis, the physician and physical therapist did not agree that a left prosthesis was indicated in this case.

"At the first team meeting, we found out that the physical therapist apparently had tried to have Mrs. Cooper 'hop' between the parallel bars during the first few days of admission and she hadn't been able to hold herself up. I pointed out that Mrs. Cooper had lost some more fluid weight (10 pounds) in the last week and her congestive heart failure was more stable. Her endurance and strength had increased since then, too. I thought it was worthwhile to try the parallel bars again."

Within a few days Mrs. Cooper was hopping up and down the parallel bars, even though her right prosthesis remained awkward-looking. After this success, the physician finally agreed to order a consultation with a prosthetist. When the prosthetist attended the meeting, the team agreed that Mrs. Cooper was a prosthetic candidate.

"I called the prosthetist a few days later to ask his opinion of Mrs. Cooper's right prosthesis because she was still having problems with it. Transfers were dangerous at times because she had to bear weight on an unstable prosthesis. The prosthetist said he hadn't been made aware of any right prosthesis problems, but that he'd assess the situation.

"Three days later, as I was helping Mrs. Cooper off the toilet, her right leg came out of the prosthesis and I just managed to ease her to the floor. I immediately called the physical therapist, who told me she just changed the stump socks again that morning. This was obviously not enough. . . .

"The next day the prosthetist adjusted the straps on Mrs. Cooper's right prosthesis. This worked for two or three days, but the 10-year-old straps stretched again and the problems continued. . . . Still, I was told repeatedly by other team members that 'there's nothing that can be done' and 'it's normal for this patient.' I knew this wasn't true, but in their opinion I was 'just the nurse, so I didn't know prosthetics.' I continued to document my assessments as well as Mrs. Cooper's persistent complaints that the right prosthesis was 'loose-fitting' and 'not right.'

"Despite all this, Mrs. Cooper was walking 40 feet in therapy on both prostheses with a walker. Physical therapy and the physician's notes indicated 'remarkable' and 'amazing' progress. But it wasn't at all surprising to me."

During week five of Mrs. Cooper's stay I did my biweekly duty of bringing up the right prosthesis fit problems with her physician. This time, however, I was told "It's being taken care of." The occupational therapists confirmed that they'd participated in a conversation with the prosthetist, physician, and the physical therapist about replacing the right prosthesis.

"When I told Mrs. Cooper that she was going to get a new right prosthesis, she was quiet for a few moments. Then she turned to me and said, 'Course you been sayin' that ever since we met.' Within two days Mrs. Cooper had a brand new right prosthesis. Soon she was walking 300 feet with a walker."

Why go to the trouble?

"I suppose this case study illustrates, once again, the problem of control and communication among health care professionals—and I'd prefer to spend my time relating positive team-building anecdotes. But more importantly, this was a powerful reminder to all of us to listen to a patient's belief in herself.

"Instead of focusing on Mrs. Cooper's deficits, the occupational therapists, the staff nurses, and I chose to focus on her many strengths. Her iron-willed determination and good humor were our greatest assets. We were amply rewarded. I'm pleased that I was able to play an instrumental role in improving the quality of life for this patient.

"What happened to Mrs. Cooper? After her two-week postdischarge appointment with her physician, Mrs. Cooper, using a walker, came to see me—with her beloved grandbabies in tow." (Smith 1993, 43–44).

This story portrays the nurse's in-between stance and the nurse's role in fighting for care that fosters the patient's well-being, even against strong opposition and mistaken judgments from the patient's physician and physical therapist. It shows how a nurse can take a strong stance concerning patient treatment in opposition to other health care professionals but, at the same time, foster cooperative teamwork. It also demonstrates why once-and-for-all decisions are often inadequate and why a series of decisions and actions is required in light of changing understanding and circumstances. It shows how intuitive judgment that includes such factors as a patient's strength and determination can be the basis for an "as if" treatment that fosters the patient's well-being. In this case, Margie Smith is a morally good nurse because her concern for the well-being of the patient is embodied in efficient, effective, and attentive nursing that eventuates in successful therapy for Mrs. Cooper. Margie's concern is not for the abstract autonomous rights of the patient. She is concerned for the personal well-being of Mrs. Cooper whom she knows well. She is so engrossed in Mrs. Cooper's situation that she knows what Mrs. Cooper wants and is capable of doing. Her personal relationship with the patient is not an add-on; it is integrally related to patient care.

Good Nurses, Not the Good Nurse

Margie is a good nurse. She is *a* good nurse, not *the* good nurse. We originally planned to discuss *the* good nurse in this chapter. But there is no *the* nurse. There is only Margie and other nurses whose outstanding ways of being mark them as good nurses. Therefore, we have discussed the meaning of being *a* good nurse rather than *the* good nurse. I am a good nurse when my concern for patients is integrally related to efficient, effective, and attentive care that fosters the well-being of my patient. Even when I am not directly concerned about my patients' well-being, I am focused on ways of fostering their well-being because I am engaged in a practice with an inherent moral sense. The moral sense of nursing practice integrally relates concern with practical know-how. Margie discloses the meaning of being a good nurse by the way in which her effective, efficient, and attentive care are integrally related to her concern for the well-being of Mrs. Cooper.

Study Questions

1. What is the primary thesis of this chapter? How is this thesis related to the nature of a practice?
2. Why do Anne and Jack contend that nursing practice is distorted when the practical aspects of nursing are divorced from the personal? Do you agree? Why or why not?
3. Why is the nurse's action in ordering a test for blood glucose level an example of outstanding nursing? Why is it also an example of outstanding moral action? What would the nurse have disclosed as the meaning of nursing and morality by playing it safe?
4. Jack and Anne contend that burnout often occurs when nurses lose the moral sense of nursing. They give the example of the nurse giving mouth-to-mouth respiration to support this contention. Does this example prove their contention, disclose the meaning of their contention, or prove that competent care is necessary? Why or why not?

5. Evaluate the movement from competence to excellence in ethics as Dreyfus and Dreyfus develop it. You may want to compare it to Benner's treatment of the movement from competence to excellence in nursing (Benner 1984). According to Anne and Jack, how are the two related?

6. What is meant by acting "as if" in nursing? Do you believe that nurses have a moral obligation to act "as if"? If so, under what circumstances?

7. What are Anne and Jack trying to disclose in the example of the nurse who let her patient sleep? Do you agree with their interpretation? Why or why not? Can you give a different or a further interpretation of the case?

8. Why do Anne and Jack believe that the in-between stance is essential in nursing care and a privileged position for making moral decisions? Do you agree? Why or why not?

9. Describe and interpret how most of the major themes of this chapter are disclosed in the case of Margie Smith. Could you also treat the same themes by discussing why Margie Smith is a good nurse? Why or why not?

10. Why did Anne and Jack call this chapter "On Being a Good Nurse" rather than "The Good Nurse"? Some philosophers argue that you could not know the meaning of being a good nurse without knowing what constitutes "the good nurse." Do you agree with Anne and Jack or with the advocates of "the good nurse"? Why?

References

Benner, Patricia. (1984). *From Novice to Expert: Excellence and Power in Clinical Nursing Practice*. Menlo Park, Cal.: Addison-Wesley.

Benner, Patricia, and Judith Wrubel. (1989). *The Primacy of Caring: Stress and Coping in Health and Disease*. Menlo Park, Cal.: Addison-Wesley.

Bishop, Anne H., and John R. Scudder, Jr. (1990). *The Practical, Moral, and Personal Sense of Nursing: A Phenomenological Philosophy of Practice*. Albany, N.Y.: State University of New York Press.

Bishop, Anne H., and John R. Scudder, Jr. (1990). *Nursing: The Practice of Caring*. New York: National League for Nursing Press.

Dreyfus, Hubert L., and Stuart E. Dreyfus. (1991). Towards a Phenomenology of Ethical Expertise. *Human Studies* 14:229–250.

Gadamer, Hans-Georg. (1981). *Reason in the Age of Science* . trans. F. G. Lawrence. Cambridge, Mass.: MIT Press.

Gilligan, Carol. (1982). *In a Different Voice: Psychological Theory and Women's Development*. Cambridge, Mass.: Harvard University Press.

Paget, Marianne A. (1988). *The Unity of Mistakes: A Phenomenological Interpretation of Medical Work*. Philadelphia: Temple University Press.

Smith, Margie. (1993). Two Legs to Stand On. *American Journal of Nursing* 93(12): 43–44.

3

Caring Presence

In the previous chapter, we contended that good nursing requires an integral relationship between efficient, effective, attentive care and personal caring relationships. A nurse in an integral caring relationship is experienced by patients as a caring presence. That such caring presence is often lacking in health care is evident in Richard Zaner's oft-made statement that patients want to know that those "who are taking care of them *really* care" for them (Zaner 1985, 92). This statement implies that patients receive effective and efficient care more often than they encounter caring presence. Roberta Messner (1993) reports that many studies of patient satisfaction have revealed that "patients' unmet expectations rarely have to do with competence. More often the problem is a perception of insensitivity to their needs or lack of respect for their viewpoint—in a word, caring" (38).

Caring Presence in Nursing Practice

Caring presence, like all forms of presence, is difficult to define. Its meaning, however, can be disclosed in concrete examples of nursing care, such as those collected by Ingegerd Harder.

She took care of me, she literally came very close to my body. I learned how much it means that someone really cares for my here and now comfort, for my physical well-being, which—I learned that, too—had a million positive effects on my more general well-being. She helped me with comfort and well-being.

From *The world of the hospital nurse: Nurse patient interactions—body nursing and health promotion. Illustrated by use of combined phenomenological/grounded theory approach* by Ingegard Harder. Copyright 1993. Aarhus, Danmarks Sygeplejerskehøjskole ved Aarhus Universitet, Skrift-serie fra Danmarks Sygeplejerskehøjskole 3/93, p. 172. Used with permission of Ingegard Harder, R.N., PhD.

Patients are capable of distinguishing between personable care and personal care and between being likably present and being skillfully and knowledgeably present. They associate caring presence with both personal and skillful-knowledgeable care, as Harder's study indicates.

That nurse had such a pleasant personality, she looked so kind, she was calm, she wanted me to feel comfortable, she wanted me to feel informed about what was happening. She was sort of 'serving' me, and she quietly organized my present world. But what about her failures, the times when she confused me, what about my feeling that she was not the most knowledgeable nurse? She left me in confusion a couple of times. But I liked her, she had a soothing effect on me. Her spontaneous warmth and calmness, I appreciated it so much.

From *The world of the hospital nurse: Nurse patient interactions—body nursing and health promotion. Illustrated by use of combined phenomenological/grounded theory approach* by Ingegard Harder. Copyright 1993. Aarhus, Danmarks Sygeplejerskehøjskole ved Aarhus Universitet, Skrift-serie fra Danmarks Sygeplejerskehøjskole 3/93, p. 172. Used with permission of Ingegard Harder, R.N., PhD.

In the above case, the patient is able to recognize that although she liked the nurse who had a pleasant personality, her nurse lacked knowledge and sometimes confused her. The patient did experience caring presence in that her nurse informed her, helped organize her world, and soothed her with warmth, kindness, and calmness. But the caring presence of a nurse requires more than being personable or even personal.

She had this efficient look about her. I did not feel rapport with her. Yet, I also knew that should things go wrong with me in some way or other, I would not mind her being on duty. She knew, she could cope in complicated situations. She made me unafraid.

From *The world of the hospital nurse: Nurse patient interactions—body nursing and health promotion. Illustrated by use of combined phenomenological/grounded theory approach* by Ingegard Harder. Copyright 1993. Aarhus, Danmarks Sygeplejerskehøjskole ved Aarhus Universitet, Skrift-serie fra Danmarks Sygeplejerskehøjskole 3/93, p. 172. Used with permission of Ingegard Harder, R.N., PhD.

In the above case, the patient recognizes the nurse's knowledge and skill as evidence of caring presence. She is not now experienced as caring presence, but should the situation require it, the patient is certain that the nurse would be there for her with effective, efficient, and attentive care. This knowledgeable and skilled nurse was not encountered by the patient as present caring presence but as potential caring presence.

Patients experience caring presence as actual or potential attending to them. As Harder observed, this quality of nursing is so essential that it often seems to the patient to have a "magical" quality. "I had a feeling that she was attending to me, even when she was not in the room for a while" (Harder, 173). In addition to patients' experiencing caring nurses as attending to them, patients recognize that caring presence combines personal concern with skilled and knowledgeable care.

It was after breakfast. I did not eat as much as I wanted to. I felt surprised, because I couldn't mobilize my will, I leaned back, as if I had used my body for hours. Suddenly she was there again, a nurse that had spent a lot of time with me the day before. She was smiling, full of energy. She went straight to the point, leaned on to the table and offered to help me have a shower in the bathroom. It seemed like climbing a mountain, but she was so convincing that I agreed. She explained the whole procedure, how she would cover the wound with plastic etc. It began sounding like heaven. I had confidence in her, she seemed to have been doing this for a hundred years. And it was heaven. Never had I thought that I would appreciate water running slowly down my body as I did that morning. I was sitting on a chair, and the nurse was next to me. I relaxed. She had a special way of offering her help in concrete ways like washing my back and my feet, which I literally could not reach that morning. "I suggest that you . . .," and "what you could do is turning your body . . .," yes she was assisting me, never taking over. I was in command, I felt. I mattered. Even though the only thing I could manage was steering the shower handle.

From *The world of the hospital nurse: Nurse patient interactions—body nursing and health promotion. Illustrated by use of combined phenomenological/grounded theory approach* by Ingegard Harder. Copyright 1993. Aarhus, Danmarks Sygeplejerskehøjskole ved Aarhus Universitet, Skrift-serie fra Danmarks Sygeplejerskehøjskole 3/93, p. 172. Used with permission of Ingegard Harder, R.N., PhD.

When we think of the knowledge and skill of nursing, we often think of high-tech situations. We chose the above example because the knowledge and skill evident in it are those of general everyday nursing care. In the above case, the knowledge and skill are so integrated with the personal care that they go unnoticed on first reading. Yet this knowledge and skill were recognized immediately by the patient as an integral ingredient in the liberating and comforting caring presence of her nurse.

Caring Presence Fosters Well-Being

Caring presence doesn't mean some emotive, sentimental, maudlin expression of feeling toward patients. It is a way of being with others that assures them of personal concern for their well-being. This way of being fosters trust, mutual concern, and positive attitudes that promote good health. When caring presence pervades a health care setting, the whole atmosphere of that setting is transformed so that not only is sound therapy fostered but patients appreciate, take pride in, and feel part of the health care endeavor. That this transformation was taking place in a free clinic was evident to one of the authors when, in the process of interviewing clients to determine their understanding of wellness and sickness, the clients continually interrupted the interview with praise and testimonials concerning the excellent care in the clinic. The following message, hand-written on a Christmas card to the staff of this clinic, expresses the attitudes of many of the clients.

Dear Folks,
Just to say you are so much a part of all of our lives. You give so much and ask so little in return. During our lifetime we are touched by many people that criss-cross our lives. But we are indeed blessed when the most caring, loving people with so much compassion in their hearts touch our hearts and life and are always there for you. Because of you very beautiful people you have made our community a better place to live.

Caring presence also supports patients facing anxiety, suffering, and death. No one ought to face pain, uncertainty, or death alone and unsupported. When patients are not supported by family and friends, nurses often offer them the support and companionship that they need. For example, nurses ensured that a two-and-one-half-year-old child, who had lived his entire life in the hospital, was not left alone.

> As the parents had become gradually less and less involved, quite naturally those who were with Johnny most often and most intimately, especially the primary-care nurses, had effectively bonded with him, to the point that they seemed even to resent the parents and took the parents' apparent lack of concern quite personally. Even the attending seemed bound up with the child in a more personal way than I had witnessed before. "Taking care of" Johnny had shifted into "caring for" Johnny. (Zaner 1993, 42)

Most people are not so alone. Many have an abundance of relatives and friends who support them with caring presence. But nurses are with patients in ways and situations that visitations to hospitals do not allow, and they have knowledge and expertise in relating to the patients that visitors do not possess. For example, a well-liked retired librarian was being visited in the hospital by another librarian and a fellow church member. She was the kind of person who had an abundance of people supporting her. When her visitors arrived, they found a woman sitting in the room who informed them that their friend was in the bathroom. Then she explained that she had been her nurse for a considerable time but had been transferred to another unit. She knew that this patient was anxious because they had been unable to find out the cause of her illness. The nurse had dropped by to inquire as to her progress and to give her support. After the patient returned and the nurse had left, the patient related how this nurse's caring presence had helped her live with the anxiety of being seriously ill without knowing why.

Caring presence often fosters the healing process itself. It often transforms the person being cared for directly. Encountering caring presence fosters the well-being of patients by transforming their way of being in the world. When giving an injection, a reassuring nurse lessens the anxiety of the patient and thus the tenseness in the muscles, thereby making the injection less painful. In most therapeutic care, lessening of tension and anxiety fosters healing and well-being. The degree to which caring presence directly fosters healing has been highly problematic in health care literature. The work of Norman Cousins (1989) with physicians and nurses, and the work of Delores Kreiger (1981) and Janet Quinn (1981) with nurses in therapeutic touch indicate that caring relationships can directly foster healing. Regardless of the degree to which healing is fostered directly by caring presence, caring presence does well fit Gilligan's definition of caring as "an activity of relationship, of seeing and responding to need, taking care of the world by sustaining the web of connection so that no one is left alone" (Gilligan 1982, 62). Not being left alone requires more than simply being attended to. It requires the personal presence of others. Thus, it affirms Zaner's contention that patients not only want to be cared for, but want to know that those who care for them really care (Zaner 1985, 96).

Harder's examples at the beginning of the chapter indicate that patients are often well aware of the ways in which caring presence is evident in nursing care. But caring presence requires a fuller articulation. Our articulation includes descriptions of personal relationships, of caring, and of presence. We will attempt this articulation assisted by the work of Martin Buber (1970), Nel Noddings (1984), and Richard Zaner (1981).

1. Buber: Personal Relations

Buber (1970) described two ways of being with others that are especially appropriate to human relationships in nursing. He contrasted personal I-Thou relationships with impersonal I-It relationships. The following case illustrates both Buber's I-It and I-Thou relationships.

Sarah is a 38-year-old woman with lymphoma. She has two young daughters, aged three and five. She has been treated for over a year by an oncologist who often has difficulty developing personal relationships with his patients. However, Sarah's intelligence and interest in participating in the decisions regarding her care have fostered a personal relationship with the seemingly distant physician.

The oncologist referred Sarah to a university medical center for a bone marrow biopsy. Securing bone marrow from Sarah in the past had proven extremely difficult because of her anatomy and bone structure. Sarah agreed to go to the medical center because of its superior diagnostic equipment, and only on condition that she would be given adequate pain medication.

Due to some unfortunate circumstance, the physician who was to perform the biopsy was unable to do so, and after a long delay, a substitute was obtained. The substitute physician not only failed to respond to Sarah's request for more pain medication but stopped the nurse from getting the medication that had been ordered by the original physician, to honor his prior agreement with Sarah. The substitute physician insisted on rigidly following what she regarded as standardized procedures for any bone marrow biopsy. After several failed attempts to get bone marrow, another physician succeeded in getting some bone marrow with great difficulty. Both physicians conducted the biopsy with standard medication and procedures, paying no attention to Sarah's request for more pain medication. In contrast, the nurse assisting with the biopsy listened attentively to Sarah's request and the reasons for making that request. Sarah later commented that the nurse was the only sensible (and sensitive) member of the biopsy team and vowed never to return to that hospital again.

After the biopsy, Sarah's husband commented to the nurse that his wife had incredible strength. The nurse expressed her agreement, having cared for Sarah during the trying, painful procedure. But the physicians who had performed the operation responded to the husband's comment with ironic disdain. They had encountered the patient as being an uncooperative patient who overreacted to pain and tried to tell them how to conduct the biopsy.

The physicians related to the patient as an It—a thing to be put in the category of uncooperative patient because she did not respond to their standardized treatment in ways that facilitated the biopsy. In contrast, the nurse responded to Sarah personally as Thou. During the biopsy, she came to know Sarah as an intelligent person who attempted to make the best of a difficult situation made worse by insensitive physicians. In her brief relationship with the patient, the nurse encountered the same person the husband knew from sharing her long and difficult struggle with cancer.

In this case incompetent behavior should not be confused with impersonal behavior. During surgical procedures competent physicians use information concerning the patient obtained from charts and interviews. Such competency does not constitute personal relationships with the patient. The nurse did secure the agreed-on pain medication by following medical orders on the chart, but her assessment of the situation came from relating to the patient in a mutually responsive way that took seriously her right to insist that the physicians give the pain medication previously agreed on and prescribed for her particular situation.

All health care workers are well aware that patients often make inappropriate suggestions about their care. Professionals are experts concerning what is best for *the patient*. But in the foregoing case, the biopsy was not done to *the patient* but to a particular person who, by working with her regular oncologist, had come to sound conclusions concerning her response to pain and the resistance of her bone structure. Although her oncologist was known for his difficulty relating to persons, he had been able to relate to Sarah personally in matters concerning her situation and treatment. The oncologist knew more than she did about cancer and treatment. But she had learned much from him in their relationship of mutual respect and shared concern for her well-being. Although her nurse during the operation was much more "personable" than her oncologist, they both related to Sarah as Thou.

In the above case, both the nurse and the oncologist are in I-Thou relationships with Sarah. I-Thou relationships concern a way of being together and not the style or the length of the relationship. For example, the nurse is personable; the oncologist is not. The nurse has known the patient only a short time and the oncologist for about a year. But in each case, Sarah is related to as a person and is responded to as she is present. Sarah is a full partner in the relationship, in that she is listened to and included in decisions about her ongoing treatment. This mutual relationship of personal response to each other is essential to all I-Thou relationships. In I-Thou relationships both partners recognize the right of each partner to his/her way of being. In I-Thou relationships, whole persons encounter each other as beings who are present to each other. Sarah related to both her physician and nurse as persons, albeit persons with special knowledge and skills encountered in special relationships. Buber recognized that, because of this imbalance, therapeutic relationships cannot be fully mutual ones, and therefore they constitute a special form of I-Thou relationships. In Sarah's relationship with her nurse and oncologist, the mutuality of their relationship is asymmetrical, but nevertheless they respond to each other as the whole person who is present in their encounter.

In contrast to the I-Thou relationships between Sarah and her oncologist and nurse, her relationship to the physicians who performed the biopsy was an I-It relationship. Instead of responding to her as a person, the physicians regarded her as a patient from whom bone marrow was to be taken. She was an uncooperative patient in that she kept insisting on more pain medication and had the audacity to question the physicians' judgment. The physicians' knowledge about biopsies and human anatomy dictated their treatment of the patient, without regard to her response to their treatment. They seemed in no way present to her suffering presence. For Buber, I-It relationships are characterized by detachment from the other, by use of knowledge about the other to categorize the other and to treat the other in a standard way, and by objectification of the otherness of the other. In an I-It relationship, there is none of the mutuality and recognition of the other that come from the reciprocal presence and personal response of I-Thou relationships.

Most nurses readily recognize I-It relationships between physicians and patients and obvious I-It relationships in nurse-patient relationships. Buber's description of I-It relationships can help nurses recognize less obvious I-It relationships in nursing, such as professionally and technically defined relationships. In I-It relationships one person detaches himself/

herself from another in order to gain knowledge that makes it possible to control the other, or, in professional language, to intervene in the life of the other. In the professional model, the nurse detaches himself/herself from the patient to consider what any competent nurse would do in these circumstances. Knowledge of good nursing comes primarily from education and is condensed in the form of maxims to be applied in situations—"in situation x the nurse does y." In this scenario, the good patient is compliant—follows the dictates of the professional nurse. The client is not present as a person but only as *the* client to be controlled by the maxims of the profession.

The technical interpretation of nursing is even more aptly described by Buber's treatment of I-It than is the professional interpretation. In the technical interpretation, the nurse is supposed to remain detached from the patient in order to meet the requirements of science. The nurse is to use knowledge obtained from scientific study to categorize and prescribe interventions to alter the patient's behavior. The patient is dealt with as an example of x to be treated by y, but not as a person.

In the foregoing, we have treated I-It relationships in nursing that tend to blind nurses to the moral and personal sense of nursing. Our treatment of these I-It relationships should not lead to the conclusion that all I-It relationships are to be avoided. Obviously, there are many situations that call for I-It relationships. Buber, in fact, contended that it is impossible to remain continually in I-Thou relationships without burning out (Buber 1970, 85). Not only is it dangerous to remain in I-Thou relationships too long, it is desirable to be in an I-It relationship to perform certain functions. Technological functions in nursing practice often require that nurses temporarily forget the person and focus on the function. This way of placing nurses in I-It relationships with patients does not mean that nurses should forget that they are working with and on fellow human beings. A way of recognizing the rights of persons in I-It relationships is needed. Buber does not give us this way, but his description of I-It and I-Thou relationships does help nurses to distinguish between the personal and the impersonal and to recognize how the impersonal can subvert the moral sense of nursing.

I-It (Thou) Relationships

A way is needed to describe impersonal relationships that support the moral and personal sense of nursing. Sally Gadow (1985) makes evident the need for such a relationship in her contention that nurses need to attend to the body object without reducing the patient to the moral status of an object (32–33). A relationship that makes it possible to deal with other persons objectively but, at the same time, to treat them with the dignity and respect due a person has been described as an I-It (Thou) relationship (Scudder and

Mickunas 1985). For example, a nurse, seeking to find a vein in an arm scarred by repeated intravenous injections and weakened by chemotherapy, needs to temporarily focus on the function rather than on the worried, suffering patient. By focusing on the function, this nurse would foster the patient's well-being by ensuring a successful procedure with minimal harm. But when focusing on the function, she/he should not forget that the patient is a person, as the parenthetical Thou indicates. I-It (Thou) describes a relationship in which a nurse can attend to the body object technically and professionally, without reducing the patient to the moral status of an object.

I-It (Thou) relationships require recognition of patient rights. If a patient says, "Stop! You're killing me," a nurse might stop, reasoning, "This is a fellow human being who has the right to decide how much pain to endure." Rights arguments are impersonal. A person has rights as a citizen, a patient, a nurse, etc., and as a fellow human being in the case of human rights. Rights are granted to individuals by impersonally placing them in categories. Being placed in the category of patient implies equal but not uniform treatment. Patients, like all human beings, are unique individuals who have a right to be treated individually. As Buber (1958) has pointed out, individuality refers to I-It relationships because individuality is determined by comparing one person with another (62). For example, the patient in the bone marrow case is different from most patients in being more susceptible to pain and having harder, thicker bones. By stressing this difference, the nurse in that case could have argued with the physicians for individualized treatment for her patient. In so doing, she would argue impersonally for individualized treatment on the grounds that her patient is a human being and therefore has the right to individualized treatment, like any other human being.

When nurses are in I-It (Thou) relationships with patients, they not only recognize patient rights but also are open to the possibility of entering into personal relationships with patients when the situation calls for it. The parentheses around the Thou indicate that the nurse maintains an awareness that this is a person, even when treating the patient impersonally. This awareness fosters the movement from the impersonal to the personal. For example, suppose in Sarah's case, the nurse is intent on treating and bandaging Sarah's wound, when suddenly Sarah turns to her and says, "How can I tell my young children that I am dying?" This calls for moving from an I-It relationship to an I-Thou relationship. It is possible that the nurse might have no better answer to the question than the patient, but, nevertheless, she should respond personally to this invitation to dialogue by entering her patient's intimate life. Her response could eventually lead her into a relationship of caring presence with a dying person—a personal relationship that one nurse has called the most fulfilling in her career (Bishop and Scudder 1990, 95–96).

Triadic Dialogue

As important as personal relationships are in nursing care, they are not the end of nursing care. Nursing care is a relationship designed to foster the well-being of the patient. One problem with Buber's interpretation of I-Thou relationships is that it describes a personal relationship with no end beyond itself, such as friendship. But nursing has an end beyond the relationship itself. Nurse-patient relationships are established to foster the well-being of one of the partners, called the patient or the client. The nurse-patient relationship is not created to develop deep personal relationships, but to foster the healing and health of the patient. The relationship between nurse and patient is intentionally therapeutic.

Fostering the well-being of patients (the moral sense of nursing) can be included in the nurse-patient relationship through triadic dialogue (Bishop and Scudder 1990). In triadic dialogue, nurse and patient respond to each other as persons, but for the purpose of fostering the well-being of the one called the patient. An excellent example of triadic dialogue was the nurse assisting a patient in taking a shower described earlier in this chapter.

> She had a special way of offering her help in concrete ways like washing my back and my feet, which I literally could not reach that morning. "I suggest that you . . .," and "what you could do is turning your body . . .," yes she was assisting me, never taking over. I was in command, I felt. I mattered. Even though the only thing I could manage was steering the shower handle. (Harder 1993, 173)

The dialogue between the nurse and patient is not only verbal but also tactile. The nurse's way of washing the patient assures the patient that eventually she will be able to wash herself, and the nurse's speech suggests how the patient can begin to bathe herself. Amazingly, this is so much the case that the patient feels she is "in command," even though she is only capable of "steering the shower handle." Even though the nurse is actually bathing the patient, the patient is already beginning self-care.

This nurse's care of her patient is an excellent example of what Martin Heidegger (1962) has called "authentic care." Authentic care empowers patients to care for themselves. In contrast, "dependent care" (our term rather than Heidegger's) takes care away from patients by making them dependent on the caregiver (Scudder 1990). Unfortunately, the term "caring presence" often connotes dependent care. But authentic caring presence empowers persons to care for themselves as much as possible.

Triadic dialogue is uniquely structured to foster authentic care. In contrast to dyadic dialogue, which focuses on the relationship of the partners and on sharing between the partners, triadic dialogue calls for fostering the well-being of one of the partners through empowerment of that partner in an I-Thou relationship. In the foregoing example, the nurse and the patient are in an I-Thou relationship that is focused on fostering the well-being of the patient by bathing her *but* in a way that teaches, that encourages and empowers her to bathe herself in the future.

2. Noddings: Caring

Nurses foster the well-being of patients through caring relationships. The description of caring by Noddings is especially appropriate to that aspect of nursing we have called caring presence. The interpretation of caring by Noddings assumes that personal relationships are "ontologically basic and the caring relation" is "ethically basic" (Noddings 1984, 150). These assumptions support the primacy of personal relationships in Buber's thought and the moral sense of those relationships in triadic dialogue. The essential meaning of caring is a relationship in which one partner fosters the well-being of the other.

Noddings describes caring in a way that makes its moral sense evident. The essential elements in a caring relationship include *"engrossment* and *motivational displacement* on the part of the one-caring and a form of *responsiveness* or *reciprocity* on the part of the cared-for" (Noddings 1984, 150). According to Noddings, the one-caring is first engrossed in the other's life and then shifts motivational concern from self to the other. She contends that when I am engrossed, "I receive the other into myself, and I see and feel with the other" (30). Thus, caring involves attempting to experience the world as the other experiences it by seeing through "the eyes of the cared-for" (13). For example, the nurse in the foregoing case concerning the bone marrow operation became engrossed in the patient's situation and was able to become present to her suffering. In contrast, the physicians were preoccupied with completing a biopsy by following routine procedures. In addition, they seemed preoccupied with their own well-being, not with that of the patient—one physician even complained to the patient during the biopsy that he would not get paid for the biopsy.

The motivational shift from the well-being of the one-caring to that of the one-cared-for is the other essential ingredient in care, as described by Noddings. In this shift, there is "displacement of interest from my own reality to the reality of the other" so that I "see the other's reality as a possibility for my own" (14). The other's possibility is fostered by taking "special regard for the particular person in a concrete situation" (24). The nurse in the bone marrow case made that motivational shift to the well-being of Sarah in her concrete situation. In contrast, the physicians in this case were not engaged in care for *this* patient; instead, they were carrying out prescribed procedures for any patient. Although the nurse's care involved professional procedures, her way of being with the patient was not primarily a professional one but a human one of caring presence.

The relationship of technical procedures to caring presence is a difficult one in contemporary health care. Physicians might well respond to our interpretation of the above case by pointing out that securing bone marrow is a technical procedure during which personal consideration needs to be excluded for the well-being of the patient. Nurses, no less than physicians, encounter the same problem. For example, the procedure of starting intravenous fluids on a person with fragile veins requires a nurse's undivided attention. Caring presence requires preoccupation with the technical when the situation calls for it. However, such temporary preoccupation does not imply that the patient is to be treated merely as a "thing" on which to conduct the procedure. Our inclusion of I-It (Thou) relationships in nurse-patient relationships describes a relationship that is essentially impersonal but in which the nurse involved in technical procedures is aware that they are being conducted on human beings. This relationship further calls for the one-caring to be open to the personal when that is called for. In the bone marrow case, this is clearly a difference between the nurse and the physicians.

In caring relationships, as described by Noddings, the one-cared-for responds to care by appreciation for care given, or by going on with his/her life in the way that care has made possible. In the bone marrow biopsy case, Sarah and her husband greatly appreciated the care of the nurse, especially since it was present in such difficult circumstances. This appreciation was deeply felt even though the nurse was not in a position to change the way that the procedure was conducted.

In addition to describing care as engrossment, motivational shift, and patient response, Noddings makes a distinction between natural caring and ethical caring that is significant for nursing practice, and especially for nursing ethics. Natural caring is "that relationship in which we respond as one-caring out of love or natural inclination" (Noddings 1984, 5). We enter into a relationship of natural caring when "we accept the natural impulse to act on behalf of the present other" (83). Presumably, the nursing scholar mentioned in Chapter 1, who said that nurses feel guilty when we point out the moral sense of nursing, meant that nurses can't always operate on the basis of natural caring and therefore feel that they are neglecting the moral sense. Nurses cannot always, and perhaps cannot usually, act out of natural caring. This dilemma of having to care, in the absence of natural caring, can be resolved through Noddings's distinction between natural caring and ethical caring. Noddings contended that when we are not motivated by natural caring, we can care because we want to be caring persons. The desire to be a caring person is motivated and empowered by appreciative remembrance of having been cared for by others.

When ethical caring is applied to nursing, nurses care out of the desire to be caring nurses, rather than out of natural care. But does this not assign a higher priority to caring out of a desire to be a caring nurse than to natural caring? It would do so for nurses for whom being a caring nurse means following the prescriptive maxims of what they have been taught nurses should do. However, if nursing is essentially caring, then being a caring nurse requires placing caring for patients above all other values. This would mean placing wanting to care for patients above loyalty to nursing, if that choice could be made. In nursing practice, being a caring nurse and valuing caring are so integrally related that such separation would be artificial and lead to inauthentic nursing. When nurses are motivated by ethical caring, they do what they do because they value caring for persons, even those persons for whom they do not naturally care. For example, when a nurse did not naturally care for an obnoxious patient, she/he would care for that patient out of the desire to be a caring person, but one who cares in the way that nurses care.

Although Noddings's interpretation of caring contributes much to the understanding of nursing care, it should be tested by being placed in the context of nursing practice. Placing it in this context will show that her interpretation of care needs (1) to include natural caring in the ethical, (2) to consider competing moral desires and limited time, and (3) to recognize the caring in practice.

Natural Caring in the Ethical

Noddings reserves the term "ethical" for caring that is done out of the desire to be a caring person, rather than out of natural caring. She makes clear that ethical caring does not have a higher priority than natural caring. For her, natural caring is preferable to ethical caring. The implication of this interpretation of caring for nursing is that nurses should care naturally when possible, but when natural care is not possible, then they should care ethically. For example, a nurse who does not naturally care for an obnoxious patient should do so because she/he wants to be a caring nurse. But to be caring, the nurse would have to become engrossed in the patient's situation and shift concern from self to the patient. Since this shift requires the nurse to shift concern for herself/himself—being a caring nurse—to the well-being of the patient, she/he cannot become a caring nurse by *seeking* to be a caring nurse, but only by seeking the well-being of clients. Consequently, desiring to be a caring nurse may initiate care for the other, but a nurse is a caring nurse only when she/he attempts to foster the well-being of others, thus fulfilling the moral sense of nursing.

There is a possible interpretation of Noddings that eliminates the shift from self—I want to be a caring person—to actual caring—being engrossed in and acting to promote another's well-being. Although Noddings usually says that in ethical caring, I care because I want to be a good person, she also says that ethical caring arises out of valuing caring itself. Ethical caring arises from "an evaluation of the caring relationship as good, as better than, superior to, other forms of relatedness. . . . The source of my obligation [to care] is the value I place on the relatedness of caring" (Noddings, 83–84). Here Noddings seems to say that I am obligated to care when I recognize the worth of caring relationships. But even so, to enter into a caring relationship, I would have to refocus my attention and effort from the worth of caring to engrossment with and actual care for the person who needed my care.

Interpreting ethical caring as caring done out of recognition of the worth of caring, rather than out of the desire to be a caring person, lessens the tension between natural caring and ethical caring. But it does not explain why caring out of natural care is not designated ethical caring, while caring out of recognition for the worth of care or the desire to be a caring person is designated as ethical. Noddings's reasoning may be that if I care for someone because I desire to, then my action has no ethical merit. However, if I care for someone because I want to be a caring person, in opposition to my natural inclinations, then my actions are virtuous or meritorious. She contends that when the remembrance of having been cared for "sweeps over us as a feeling—as an 'I must'—in response to the plight of the other," it encounters a "conflicting desire to serve our own interests" (Noddings 1984, 79–80). Since ethical caring is marked by conflicting desires, it "requires an effort that is not needed in natural caring" (80). Therefore, in order to be ethical, according to Noddings, I must choose to act against my natural inclinations by caring for those I do not naturally care for—because I value caring. Noddings seems to believe that an action can be designated as ethical only when a person is forced to choose to act morally against natural desires. Hence, for Noddings, acting out of natural caring cannot be called ethical. This reasoning could lead to the odd conclusion that nurses can be ethical only when they do not care naturally for any of their patients. We can escape this outlandish conclusion by interpreting the ethical to include actions done both out of natural caring and out of the desire to be a caring person. Thus, nursing ethics would include fostering the well-being of clients out of natural caring as well as out of the desire to be a caring nurse.

Conflicting Moral Desires and Limited Time

Why inclusion of natural caring in the ethical is appropriate in nursing can be shown by considering dilemmas nurses face that fall outside of the context of Noddings's natural caring versus ethical caring. In contending that ethical caring "requires an effort that is not needed in natural caring" (80), Noddings fails to consider moral tensions faced in natural caring that require considerable moral effort. One such effort occurs when nurses, in natural caring, find themselves torn between care for patient and self. A nurse completing an understaffed night shift, her body aching and exhausted and her nerves on edge, feels a natural desire to care for a patient who especially needs her care. The nurse faces a moral choice between a natural desire to care for the patient and a natural desire to care for self. It took Nurse Echo Heron many exhausting years filled with tension to learn that those who care for others must care for themselves (Heron 1987).

In nursing practice, nurses can and often do naturally care for persons in circumstances that force them to make moral choices due to limited time. For example, at the end of his/her shift, a nurse faces several situations involving natural caring. One patient who is several hours post-operative needs to be catheterized; another patient is experiencing severe post-operative pain, and no post-operative orders have been written; a third patient is quite anxious about going home because no one is at home to help her after discharge. The nurse naturally cares for each of these persons and, therefore, would like, if time permitted, to care for each of them. Unfortunately, time to care for all three is lacking. The nurse is faced with choosing between the urgent needs to catheterize and to get an order for pain medication and the need to counsel a patient with whom she/he has developed a special relationship. The nurse reasons that the next nurse probably would not have the special relationship but could do the catheterization and call the physician for the order. Requiring the first two patients to wait, however, would prolong their suffering. We give this example to show that moral dilemmas in nursing are not limited to situations in which the alternative is between natural care and ethical care. It further illustrates that moral choice is needed when nurses feel compelled by natural caring to care for different patients, but have limited time. The pressure of time is almost always present in concrete moral situations but is often ignored in abstract discussions of moral decision making.

Those who care for others often face the moral dilemma of choosing for whom to care given limited time. For this reason, Martha Nussbaum contends that to "be a good human being is to have a kind of openness to the world . . . . a willingness to be exposed" (Moyers 1989, 448). Nussbaum contends that good persons are open to and expose themselves to caring relationships, knowing that they will be led to grief and tragedy as well as to fulfillment. Nussbaum claims that traditional ethics seeks to solve moral problems in a clear-cut and certain manner. Traditional ethics achieves its clarity and certainty by falsifying the complexity of moral situations (Nussbaum 1986, 343–372). Nurses are continually thrust into caring relationships in complex situations with time limitations that inherently involve both tragedy and fulfillment. Remaining open and exposed are moral imperatives for all who answer the call to care.

Caring in Practice

Noddings limits her treatment of caring to the subjective side of encounters with others. I care for others when I am engrossed in their situation and shift my concern from my well-being to their well-being. This shift of concern does require me to act. I "must act to eliminate the intolerable, to reduce the pain, to fill the need, to actualize the dream" (Noddings 1984, 14). But in order to act to eliminate the intolerable, reduce the pain, fill the need, and actualize the dream, I need empowerment. In nursing, empowerment comes from appropriating the practice of nursing. When authentically appropriated, nursing practice becomes empowering possibilities rather than traditional directives. The practice of nursing empowers nurses to care, but it does not make choices concerning care for them.

Empowered action requires more than caring out of natural or ethical concern for the patient. The empowerment of nursing practice fits that aspect of being that Heidegger labeled "ready-to-hand," in that past practitioners have left us ways of caring for the ill and debilitated and of fostering healthy being. Nurses care for patients by appropriating these "ready" ways to care. That Noddings missed this aspect of care is evident in her treatment of practice in education, her field of expertise. For her, practice merely means learning how to care by doing it. She seems not to grasp the meaning of practice, much less the significance of its inherent moral sense for ethics. For this reason, she cannot call natural caring ethical. If ethics in nursing concerns fulfilling its moral sense, however, then when the nurse acts to fulfill that sense, he/she is being moral whether acting out of natural caring or out of the desire to be a caring person. Natural caring appears to be more desirable than ethical caring because it directly fosters the well-being of the ill and debilitated rather than requiring a refocusing from concern for self—desiring to be a caring nurse or valuing caring itself—to concern for the well-being of the patient. Ethical caring would seem to be supplementary to natural caring, in that it would come into play only when natural care was not adequate. Put positively, a morally good nurse would foster the well-being of patients as an act of natural caring whenever possible, but when a nurse did not care naturally, he/she would care out of ethical caring. Ethical caring would require a shift from valuing caring or from wanting to be a caring nurse to concern for fostering the well-being of patients. This shift from self to other is called for by nursing practice—its inherent moral sense requires caring relationships that foster the well-being of others.

Regardless of whether nurses care for patients naturally or out of the desire to be caring nurses, they should not separate the practice of caring from the subjective meaning of care. Separation of motive from action artificially separates care as concern from care as practice. Noddings's description of care as engrossment and motivational shift is an excellent description of the subjective experience of caring. This description does not refer to inner motivation that "causes" caring practice. It merely describes the subjective side of the integral relationship between care (concern) for patients and care (practice) of patients.

The care *for* patients and the care *of* patients are integrally related in nursing practice. In a practice, meaning is implicit in doing. Consequently, subjective concern for patients often grows out of the experience of caring practice. The meaning of caring progressively informs practice as nurses learn care (concern) by engaging in caring (practice).

Learning meaning by participation in human activities is one of the primary ways that human beings learn. Remy Kwant (1965) describes how meaning develops in children in a way that suggests how the meaning of caring develops.

> We can verify all this when we observe how a child begins to act. He grows up in a house as in a little manipulable world, in which things are handled by the other occupants of the house. The child sees these persons act and in their actions the meaning of the things is activated, brought to light. He begins to imitate and through imitation gradually makes his own the meaning which things have for the others. Thus he begins to act as a human being. The child sees in the actions of the others the realization of his own possibilities. In the same way he learns to speak. The child grows up in a speaking community. He imitates the sounds, appropriates the words and gradually begins to live in the meaning of these words. (Kwant 1965, 81)

Noddings's belief that caring develops in the above manner is evident when she says, "I have a picture of those moments in which I was cared for and in which I cared, and I may reach toward this memory and guide my conduct by it" (Noddings 1984, 80). For Noddings, becoming a caring presence depends on having experienced being cared for and having cared for others.

Ways of caring are passed on to new generations through human creations. How this care is evident in human habitations is made clear by Erazim Kohák.

> It is a sense of a presence such as humans experience on entering a home in the dweller's absence. Unlike the abandoned, looted dwellings left in the wake of revolutions or the gutted shells of the inner city, . . . a dwelling, though empty, feels cared for, as if there were a cherishing and a rightness. The house *belongs:* on entering it, we sense its order not simply as an order, but specifically as the order of a *Lebenswelt,* of an inhabited context ordered by a caring presence. (Kohak 1984, 189)

In similar manner, the caring presence of those who have cared for the well-being of others before us inhabits the practice of nursing that we have inherited. We become nurses by inhabiting and appropriating their way of being in our care for patients.

Nancy Diekelmann (1990) attempts to teach nurses the meaning of caring by engaging in dialogue with them concerning the meaning of their practice. She does not assume that they are already motivated to care and need only to learn how. Instead, Diekelmann attempts through dialogue to make evident the care (concern) that is inherently present in practice. The question about whether care (concern) comes prior to practice and motivates it, or comes out of the experience of caring (practice), is a major issue only to those who make the artificial separation of motive from action. To those who reject this artificial separation, it is enough to say that care (concern) and care (practice) are so integrally related to each other that it is impossible and unimportant to say which comes first. It is possible, however, to identify engrossment and motivational shift as an integral aspect of nursing care. Patients refer to this subjective side of nursing care when they say that they want to know that the nurse who cares for them really cares for them. But engrossment and motivational shift are not experienced apart from practice but in and through the practice of caring.

3. Zaner: Caring Response to Presence

Noddings's treatment of care and Zaner's treatment of presence (Zaner 1981) can be formulated into an interpretation of caring presence especially significant for nursing ethics. Zaner places more stress on the response of others and on responsibility for others than does Noddings. Whereas Noddings focuses on describing the experience of the one-caring as engrossment and motivational shift, Zaner focuses on describing the meeting of self and other as vivid presence and co-presence. In describing that meeting, he gives much more attention than Noddings to how the one-cared-for experiences the one-caring. In his description, the one-caring is experienced as available and empowering by the one-cared-for.

We will explore the meaning of caring presence by looking at it in light of Zaner's treatment of (1) reflexive presence to the lived body, (2) vivid presence, and (3) co-presence. We say "in light of his treatment" because it is not our purpose to fully explicate his treatment of these themes as they are developed in his book *The Context of Self* (1981). His treatment has generated our thought concerning caring presence, and that thought has been further enhanced by personal dialogue with him concerning the meaning of presence and its implications for nursing ethics. Thus, Zaner's work has called forth a creative response from us. In response to Zaner, we first will show how Zaner's treatment of presence can enhance the understanding of nursing care. Then, by bringing Noddings's caring and Zaner's presence together, we will formulate a caring presence especially significant for nursing ethics.

Reflexive Presence to the Lived Body

Nursing requires care of the lived body. The relationship between nurse and patient is a strange one in which two partners care for the lived body of one of them. Equally odd is that although patients live their bodies, they may talk about them as if they were detached objects. They often need help from nurses to attend to and describe the experience of their lived bodies. In some cases, nurses even have to help patients learn how to relive their bodies, as we will show in the case of Mr. Jones in Chapter 5.

One difficulty in appropriating Noddings's treatment of care for nursing is that it is so exclusively oriented to interpersonal care that it almost precludes focusing on care of the lived body. Zaner's treatment of reflexive presence helps remedy this deficiency. Zaner contends that as we engage the world we can be reflexively present to our own bodies. This reflexive presence is what makes it possible for us to know our bodies as lived. Most athletes, even though they are focused on the game, are aware of their bodies as they engage in sport. For example, a physician advised an overweight, sedentary patient to take up jogging. He warned the patient about overexerting his heart and gave him instructions concerning his target heart rate and how to check his pulse while jogging. The patient invited his brother, who was 20 years older than he but quite athletic, to run with him. The younger brother ran the mile faster than his older brother, but his heart rate didn't return to normal within the expected time. In contrast, the older brother's heart rate returned to normal earlier than expected. When the younger brother asked his older brother, who was not a jogger, how he accomplished that, the older brother replied, "I listened to my body as I ran."

Most of us are not overtly conscious of our body as we live. One of the primary meanings of illness is that it forces us to attend to the lived body. We say, "My shoulder is stiff," "I can't get my breath," "My back aches," "I'm constipated." Normally I pay no attention to my shoulder as I serve an ace past my tennis opponent. I don't even say thank you to my shoulder. When my physician asks me if I have been short of breath, I say, "Yes, in the third set in a match with an opponent half my age." "Bull!" my physician retorts, acknowledging that my lungs are functioning better than would be expected in someone my age. Since our shoulders and lungs go unnoticed until they trouble us, we have difficulty in describing our experience of them to nurses and physicians. When we attempt such description, we describe them in terms of our lived body and not of the body as an anatomical object. I say, "My shoulder is stiff," not "I have a torn rotator cuff," or "I was out of breath after the first game of a very slow match," not "I am experiencing the onset of asthma." Once the asthma is diagnosed, however, I will be quite aware of the connection between my breathing and vigorous exercise. In fact, I may use it as an excuse for my inability to cover the court.

Nurses and physicians need to be able to draw out patients' experiences of their lived body. Unfortunately, physicians often, and nurses sometimes, request information about the body from patients in ways that lead patients away from their experience of their lived body. Often physicians are so focused on diagnosing disease that they carefully request experiences that will indicate the likelihood of a certain disease. Usually, some standard medical procedure based on theory controls what they ask for and what they attend to. Frequently, they dismiss unsolicited descriptions of the lived body of the patient as an irrelevant waste of their time.

The difference between using theoretical perspectives to select certain experiences of the body and eliciting the lived experience of a patient can best be shown by an example from clinical practice.

Sam was a seventy-five-year-old man with a diagnosis of emphysema. He had been to his physician several times complaining of pain. When the physician asked him where the pain was located, he rubbed an area in his lower chest region, and the physician attributed this pain to Sam's chronic lung condition. Sam complained to a nurse one day that his pain was getting worse and that the physician did not seem to know what the problem was. The nurse asked Sam to show her just exactly where the pain was. When Sam pressed on the area of the pain, it was obviously not in the lung region but in the area just below the diaphragm, where Sam had a hernia from a previous surgery. The nurse asked him to describe in detail what the pain was like and how long he had had it. It seemed to the nurse that the pain as described was likely the result of a strangulated hernia. She suggested that Sam call his physician to discuss this possibility. Sam called the physician, who arranged to see him almost immediately. Sam, however, had a coughing spell prior to seeing the physician, and the strangulation broke loose from the force of the cough. Almost immediately Sam's pain was relieved. When Sam's physician examined him, he confirmed that Sam's pain had probably resulted from a strangulated hernia.

What the physician did not know was that his diagnosis was made possible by a nurse's caring presence to Sam's lived body, rather than by medical preoccupation with symptoms that confirmed a previous diagnosis. Since nurses spend much more time than physicians with patients in ongoing relationships, they have a special responsibility to help patients learn to be reflexively present to their own lived bodies. Such presence is necessary for patients to be able to assume responsibility for their own health care.

Vivid Presence

In the foregoing examples of care for Sam and Sarah, both nurses are obviously vividly present to their patients. Zaner (1981) describes vivid presence as a relationship in which persons are present to each other and at the same time aware of their shared presence. This shared presence is brought about by each of the partners' tuning in to each other. This tuning in creates a shared common experience rather than "'two series of events,' yours and mine" (Zaner, 230). In vivid presence the partners create a common flow of experience in which each is aware of being in this shared relationship.

> We, you and I, each in our own ways, *experience our relationship itself*, ("we have a good marriage," or "we are really having fun," etc.), *as well as one another*, ("aren't you having a good time?") *and in the relationship each relates himself to himself*, ("I'm having a good time!" "So am I!") *and to the other* ("You didn't act like you were having a good time!" "Neither did you!"). (Zaner 1981, 231)

In vivid presence, we attune to each other in a way that leads us into a shared common experiencing of self in the world. The consciousness of each partner is focused on their shared world in which each person is reflexively aware of that person as being in the relationship.

In the foregoing description of vivid presence, Zaner is not focused on health care, but rather on how the self is constituted in relationships of vivid presence. We are interested in how vivid presence contributes to our understanding of nursing care. Consequently, our consideration of vivid presence will concern partners in asymmetrical relationships in which one partner is caring for the other while the other is receiving care. The implication of Zaner's vivid presence for nursing care can best be seen through an example from clinical practice. The following narrative was written by a nursing student working as a nurse extern.

While working as a nurse extern one evening, I was checking on my patients' progress with dinner trays. In one lady's room, I casually asked how she was doing with her dinner tray. She stated, 'Okay.' We said a few words and as I was on my way out the door, she said she probably wasn't very hungry because her chest was 'tight.' I was busy but stopped in my tracks and asked her to tell me about this 'tightness.' The 'tightness' turned out to be chest pain radiating to her left arm. I immediately told the charge nurse who called the physician who ordered oxygen and a medication. I stayed in the patient's room for 45 minutes monitoring her blood pressure every fifteen minutes. Suppose I hadn't asked another question?

In the foregoing example, the nurse and patient initially are not vividly present to each other. They share in a casual everyday experience of one helping the other in partaking of a meal. The presence becomes vivid when the nurse recognizes, in the patient's parting comment, an indication of impending danger. She returns to the patient, and they become vividly present to each other. The focus of their shared presence is one partner's consciousness of her body as she attempted to eat the meal. The nursing partner is able to elicit the patient's lived experience of her own body in a way that alerts the nurse to the possibility of a heart attack in progress. This occurs when the nurse shifts from the ordinary everyday experience of helping with the meal to the vivid presence that elicited the patient's description of what she was experiencing in her own body. The patient is able to share that experience because her nurse helps her recover her reflexive presence of her body as she attempted to eat the meal. Through entering into a relationship of vivid caring presence with the patient, the nurse becomes aware of herself as a nurse, not as a student nurse extern, but as a nurse in the full meaning of that term.

In the above example, preoccupation with everyday routine care could have blinded the nurse to a possible heart attack. Technological and professional ways of being with patients also can obscure the kind of care a patient needs. Vivid presence to the patient often discloses the care needed, as the following case shows.

Entering Ms. Frazier's room, I saw a frightened, angry, almost panicky woman who showed no neurological deficits other than disorientation. But she was visibly dehydrated (dry mouth, furrowed tongue, dry conjunctiva). . . . Her ankles and left wrist were anchored to the bed rails, but she'd apparently broken out of the right wrist restraint, pulled out her Foley and her IV and broken the IV board at the elbow. She was tangled in bedding and wailing loudly.

Since she had apparently been "in good health" a short while ago and because she had no history of confusion, falls, or transient ischemic attacks, I decided to leave the catheter out and offer her PO fluids. Immediately, she drank 10 ounces of water and four ounces of apple juice, so I left the IV out as well.

Speaking calmly, I quieted Ms. Frazier, helped her sit up at the bedside, and changed her bedding. She didn't want to go back to bed, but I calmed her and sang her to sleep with lullabies and smooth strokes along her hands, arms, cheeks, and forehead.

During the night, I made sure Ms. Frazier was roused hourly for fluids, toileting, and neurological checks. By morning shift report, she had an intake of 1,350 ml, an output of 900 ml, and was oriented and talking with anticipation about going home. She said she felt better and told us about her fall and how she'd had less than usual to drink the previous week because she'd been having a problem with urinary frequency.

Ms. Frazier was discharged home that afternoon under the watchful eye of her son and with a prescription for trimethoprim/ sulfamethoxazole (Septra) and a mini-lecture on the importance of drinking enough fluids. All her neurological tests were negative.

A week later, the night-shift supervisor formally reprimanded me for not following the physician's orders, especially concerning the IV and Haldol. Apparently one of the physicians had gone straight to her to complain . . . without talking to me about the patient first.

I managed to convince the nursing supervisor that the situation did not warrant waking the intern and that my assessment of the patient had been accurate. I felt frustrated that my role as nurse was still perceived as that of handmaiden/babysitter. I was angry that anyone could be treated as Ms. Frazier had been. . . .

In Ms Frazier's case, the supervisor and the physician were focusing on acute care technologies, rather than on the unique, frightened, confused woman I saw. (Ball 1989, 1466–1467)

The nurse in this example is vividly present to Ms. Frazier and her situation. Her immediate response was not to the broken wrist restraint, the pulled-out catheter, nor the pulled-out IV but to the "frightened, angry, almost panicky woman." The response of the physicians in the Emergency Department to this patient apparently had been to use the technological treatments of intravenous fluids and Foley catheter. The nurse, in contrast, had begun with the vivid presence of the patient and from their relationship concluded that the simpler, more direct treatment of oral fluids was indicated. In addition, her personal comforting relationship with the patient made restraining unnecessary, understanding the patient's situation possible, and giving oral fluids an option. In short, her vivid caring presence to this unique person in a particular situation enabled her to give excellent nursing care.

Vivid presence is important in health care because, as Zaner (1981) points out, "in the bulk of our face-to-face relations, we are most often merely 'facing' one another as relative strangers, as relatively typified . . . and anonymous" (232). This is often the case with nurses and patients who are assigned to each other. In the foregoing example of the nursing student, she became vividly present to her patient whom she hardly knew. Further, the nature of her vivid presence to the patient required that the patient be reflexively present to her body so that she could describe to the nurse what she experienced. In the second example, the nurse's vivid presence to an unknown patient led to appropriate care that challenged the physician's technological response and treatment.

Co-presence

Vivid presence is distinct from co-presence, according to Zaner (1981). This distinction is crucial in health care because vivid presence stresses reciprocal relationships between unique individuals, whereas co-presence stresses a mutual relationship with knowledge of the other and some degree of intimacy. Co-presence involves a mutual relationship in which both persons are present to each other as persons. In co-presence the partners form an intimate relationship in which they "make music together" (Zaner 1981, 236).

Making music together requires the partners to empower each other. Empowering each other is, for Zaner, essential to any mutual relationship. Mutual empowerment fosters freedom: "the encouraging, enabling, empowering of self to be precisely *its own self* in mutuality with the other self, which is a *potency*. That potency is . . . *freedom*" (234). But giving in a mutual relationship requires "being able *to receive* the other's giving" (234).

Receiving the other's giving requires knowing of the other's availability. Zaner regards availability as the essence of we-relationships. We-relationships are "experienced by each as a being—available—to one another" (232). Caring relationships, obviously, require such availability. One of Zaner's most important contributions to nursing is the recognition that availability is essential to caring presence. Patients experience nurses' caring presence through their availability.

Although availability and empowerment are essential to caring presence, availability is more often associated with relationships of caring presence than is empowerment. Benner is distressed by the dissociation of empowerment from caring. She says, "I am concerned when I hear nurses say that the very qualities essential to their caring role are the source of their powerlessness in the male-dominated hospital hierarchy" (Benner 1984, 207). For her, as well as Zaner, all caring relationships require empowerment.

Zaner's co-presence, with its stress on empowering relationships and availability, expands our understanding of care. Caring does, as Noddings contends, involve engrossment with the experience of others and motivational shift in which we act to foster the other's well-being. But such action does require empowerment. Nurses care by acting on behalf of patients and by enabling them to care for themselves. Both types of care require nurses to be available to patients and to make that availability known. But available caring presence that fosters authentic care requires mutual empowerment that frees the patient for self-care. Combining Zaner's sense of co-presence with Noddings's sense of caring would entail a motivational shift that empowers the other to be as self-directing as possible.

Concluding Exemplar

The exemplar we have chosen to disclose the meaning of caring co-presence also serves as a concrete summary of the chapter. It discloses the meaning of availability, of empowerment, of engrossment, of motivational shift, of I-Thou relationships, and of triadic dialogue.

After listening to the physician's report, I began to realize that Midori was dying. My own sadness and fear were less important than my being with her.

Entering her room, I sat at the edge of Midori's bed. Her breathing was shallow and rapid. With each labored breath, her neck muscles strained and her abdomen protruded. We looked at each other, searching for the right thing to say. Only our tears came. Then silence.

"Before I die, I just want to go home, pack my things, and clean up my room so my family won't have to worry about it. I just want to spend a couple of weeks with them, without their knowing that I will die soon."

Her eyes focused downward as she clutched at the bed sheet. "To be honest, I would rather die while under anesthesia than suffocate to death."

Then she looked at me. "I am being selfish, burdening you with all of this. I should be strong."

"You are such a beautiful person," I told her. Then again we sat in silence and tears.

The next morning, I was relieved to see her resting comfortably, breathing with little difficulty. During the day, she had many visitors. She had asked me earlier not to mention to anyone the seriousness of her condition. She seemed to forget the gravity of her prognosis as she unselfishly entertained her friends and family.

I went in to check on her after all had left.

"All my friends are so wonderful," she said. "They all care about me so much. I told them I was going home tomorrow. I didn't tell them everything."

She gathered her energy and asked me to help her wash up and take a walk. As we stood together at the mirrored basin, I saw the reflection of her small contorted body. She stood less than five feet tall—her spinal column curved to the right, an adaptation her body had made over the years, allowing her to breathe more easily. I reached for the warm, soapy washcloth and gently scrubbed her back. I could feel Midori beginning to relax as the water cleansed her body. Glancing at her reflection in the mirror, I saw a woman who suddenly looked so frail and helpless. Her body was straining, using every means to survive.

The hospital I work at is an enormous, overgrown monster—towers of steel and concrete with endless labyrinths of hallways and people scurrying in every direction. There is one place of solace, however, where a large window overlooks the city. During the day, it is like any other window, offering a view of the city's architecture, traffic, pedestrians, and an occasional helicopter. At night, however, it becomes a magical opening into the darkness where a thousand lights come alive.

I suggested to Midori that we take a walk to the window as the sun was beginning to set. Her eyes lit up when she saw the view.

"How beautiful!" she sighed.

I put my arm around her, holding her close, protecting her. I knew that this was the one place Midori could leave her illness behind.

"I just hope to go home and spend a few weeks with my family and friends."

I held her tighter.

"You know," she said, "these last two days have been the most important days of my life. I am grateful that you have helped me through them."

I left the hospital that night overwhelmed by the impact this woman had made on my life. She helped me to see nursing from a new perspective. We all get caught up in the daily routines of nursing—giving drugs, changing linens, charting. After six years in nursing, I suddenly realized what it *really* meant to be a nurse. (Dyck 1989, 825)

The meaning of being a nurse for Beverly is to be a caring presence to her patient. In the above case, caring presence is dialogical—that is, fully personal in the sense of Buber's I-Thou—but the dialogue is triadic in that it seeks to foster the well-being of Midori. Beverly is engrossed in her patient's situation and makes the motivational shift. She describes this shift. "My own sadness and fear were less important than my being with her." She is not only vividly co-present with her patient, but her availability invites Midori into a very intimate co-presence. Midori is empowered through caring presence in the subtle and inconspicuous ways typical of such empowerment. Her caring relationship with Beverly helps empower her to decide to live the rest of her life with her family rather than undergo a very dangerous surgery that could take her life or leave her on a ventilator for the rest of her life. Their relationship, and especially viewing the city together, helps integrate her living and dying. Beverly's caring presence supports Midori's life-affirming way of being, in the face of imminent death. From their relationship of caring co-presence with each other, Midori could say, "You know these last two days have been the most important days of my life. I am grateful that you have helped me through them," and Beverly could realize "what it *really* meant to be a nurse."

Study Questions

1. What do the examples of caring given by Ingegerd Harder disclose about the meaning of caring presence?
2. What contributions do Anne and Jack believe caring presence can make to well-being? Give other examples of ways in which caring presence fosters well-being.
3. Using the example of Sarah, describe and contrast I-It and I-Thou relationships. Give examples of each relationship from your own experience.
4. Describe an I-It (Thou) relationship. Why should nurses establish I-It(Thou) relationships with patients rather than I-It relationships?
5. Describe in your own words what Noddings means by a caring relationship. Give your own examples of caring relationships in nursing.
6. What implications does Noddings's distinction between natural caring and ethical caring have for nursing care? How does "ethical caring" answer the problem of caring for those for whom nurses do not naturally care?
7. Why should the ethical include both natural caring and ethical caring?
8. Why must limited time be considered in making moral decisions concerning for whom to care?
9. Why should nursing care include empowerment by appropriating the practice of nursing as well as caring out of natural and ethical caring? Why is it artificial to separate caring as concern from caring as practice?
10. In a small group setting, discuss the ways that nursing students can learn the meaning of caring and how to care.
11. Describe some ways that nurses can help patients to be reflexively aware of their bodies.
12. Using the examples in the book, discuss the meaning of vivid presence. Describe an experience of vivid presence that you have had with a patient. Why are relationships of vivid presence needed in nursing care?
13. By interpreting the care of Midori, discuss the meaning of caring co-presence. Why are availability and empowerment necessary in relationships of co-presence?
14. Discuss the adequacy of Anne and Jack's interpretation of the relationship of Beverly and Midori as a summary of caring presence.
15. Anne and Jack were deeply moved by reading of the relationship between Beverly and Midori. Do you believe that moving stories of caring presence make significant contributions to understanding nursing ethics? Why or why not?

References

Ball, Barbara L. (1989). When the Cure is Caring. *American Journal of Nursing* 89:1466–1467.

Benner, Patricia. (1984). *From Novice to Expert: Excellence and Power in Clinical Nursing Practice.* Menlo Park, Cal.: Addison-Wesley.

Bishop, Anne H., and John R. Scudder, Jr. (1990). *The Practical, Moral, and Personal Sense of Nursing: A Phenomenological Philosophy of Practice.* Albany, N.Y. : State University of New York Press.

Buber, Martin. [ca. 1923] (1958). *I and Thou.* 2nd ed. trans. R. G. Smith. New York: Charles Scribner's Sons.

Buber, Martin. [ca. 1923] (1970). *I and Thou.* trans. W. Kaufmann. New York: Charles Scribner's Sons.

Cousins, Norman. (1989). *Head First: The Biology of Hope.* New York: E. P. Dutton.

Diekelmann, Nancy. (1990). Nursing Education: Caring, Dialogue, and Practice. *Journal of Nursing Education* 29:300–305.

Dyck, Beverly. (1989). The Paper Crane. *American Journal of Nursing* 89:824–825.

Gadow, Sally. (1985). Nurse and Patient: The Caring Relationship. In *Caring, Curing, Coping: Nurse, Physician, Patient Relationships,* eds. Anne H. Bishop and John R. Scudder, Jr. University, Ala.: University of Alabama Press.

Gilligan, Carol. (1982). *In a Different Voice: Psychological Theory and Women's Development.* Cambridge, Mass.: Harvard University Press.

Harder, Ingegerd. (1993). *The World of the Hospital Nurse: Nurse Patient Interactions—Body Nursing and Health Promotion. Illustrated by Use of a Combined Phenomenological/Grounded Theory Approach.* Aarhus, Danmarks Sygeplejerskehøjskole ved Aarhus Universitet, Skrift-serie fra Danmarks Sygeplejerskehøjskole.

Heidegger, Martin. (1962). *Being and Time.* trans. J. Macquarrie and E. Robinson. New York: Harper and Row.

Heron, Echo. (1987). *Intensive Care: The Story of a Nurse.* New York: Ballantine.

Kohák, Erazim. (1984). *The Embers and the Stars: A Philosophical Inquiry into the Moral Sense of Nature.* Chicago: University of Chicago Press.

Kreiger, Delores. (1981). *Foundations of Holistic Health Nursing Practices: The Renaissance Nurse.* Philadelphia: J. B. Lippincott.

Kwant, Remy C. (1965). *Phenomenology of Social Existence.* Pittsburgh: Duquesne University Press.

Messner, Roberta L. (1993). What Patients *Really* Want from Their Nurses. *American Journal of Nursing* 93(8): 38–41.

Moyers, Bill. (1989). *A World of Ideas.* New York: Doubleday.

Noddings, Nel. (1984). *Caring: A Feminine Approach to Ethics and Moral Education.* Berkeley: University of California Press.

Nussbaum, Martha C. (1986). *The Fragility of Goodness: Luck and Ethics in Greek Tragedy and Philosophy.* Cambridge: Cambridge University Press.

Quinn, Janet. (1981). Client Care and Nurse Involvement in a Holistic Framework. In *Foundations of Holistic Health Nursing Practices: The Renaissance Nurse,* ed. D. Kreiger, 197–210. Philadelphia: J. B. Lippincott.

Scudder, John R., Jr. (1990). Dependent and Authentic Care: Implications of Heidegger for Nursing Care. In *The Caring Imperative in Education*, eds. M. Leininger and J. Watson, 59–75. New York: The National League for Nursing Press.

Scudder, John R., Jr., and Algis Mickunas. (1985). *Meaning, Dialogue, and Enculturation: Phenomenological Philosophy of Education*. Washington, D.C.: Center for Advanced Research in Phenomenology; University Press of America.

Zaner, Richard M. (1981). *The Context of Self: A Phenomenological Inquiry Using Medicine as a Clue*. Athens, Ohio: Ohio University Press.

Zaner, Richard M. (1985). "How the Hell Did I Get Here?" Reflections on Being a Patient. In *Caring, Curing, Coping: Nurse, Physician, Patient Relationships*, eds. Anne H. Bishop and John R. Scudder, Jr., 80–105. University, Ala.: University of Alabama Press.

Zaner, Richard M. (1993). *Troubled Voices: Stories of Ethics and Illness*. Cleveland, Ohio: Pilgrim Press.

4

Called to Care

Nurses such as Beverly Dyck (1989) and patients such as Midori call us to care. Beverly calls us to be caring persons through her example of caring. Midori calls us to care for her through her need for care, and her authentic, sensitive way of eliciting that care. In Noddings's terms, Midori calls us through natural care and Beverly through ethical care. Encountering a patient like Midori evokes natural caring. Encountering a caring person like Beverly evokes a desire to be such a person.

Evocative examples that call us to care foster integral care. Integral care is a way of being with others in which the desire to care, the purpose of care, the meaning of care, and the act of caring are one. In our time we have dismembered integral care by assigning the desire to care to psychology, the meaning of caring to philosophy, and the practice of caring to those concerned with procedures and methodology. This separation is assumed when exemplars of moral excellence are used to arouse feelings, rather than to evoke a way of being. So-called charismatic speakers—some promoters, politicians, and preachers—make their goal to manipulate the feelings of others. Listeners often respond to these speakers by feeling ennobled rather than by acting nobly. In contrast, when meaning, feelings, and actions are not separated, examples of caring call persons into caring ways of being.

Being Called to Care

Peggy Chinn (1994) contends that being called to care is an appropriate description of evoking that way of being called integral care.

> "Calling" can mean the power of naming. "A call" can mean the power of purpose. "Being called" can mean the existence that is signified by naming, as well as the fuel for action that is fired by purpose. "Called to care" is a willingness to Be in significant relation, to be responsive to others, to be in spirit together, in human existence together. In a deeply spiritual sense, it is the highest calling. In a profoundly practical sense, it is the most urgent calling beckoning all people on the earth today. (Chinn 1994, vii)

Chinn contends that interpreting care as a potential way of being into which we are called is an appropriate way of understanding caring.

> The human potential to care, like the human potential to be authentic, cannot be classified or characterized as a single "thing," nor can it conform to classifications. It cannot be boxed, packaged, or delivered on command. As a human potential, it can be envisioned, it can be imagined, it can be experienced, it can be learned, it can be nurtured. Caring can be called forth; it can be inspired. It can be called forth from any human. As a potential, it can be developed more fully as it is practiced, understood, responded to, explored, envisioned. (Chinn 1994, viii)

Caring is called forth by envisioning future possibilities for well-being. A possible future project that seems destined to foster human well-being calls us into action. In contrast to the future orientation of calling, some ethical considerations involve using a universal ethical principle to make rational judgments about moral choices that prescribe moral actions. The principle used is believed to have religious or philosophical foundations that are good for all times. Those who challenge this approach often point out the difficulty in establishing that one principle is preferable to others: for instance, in health care, the principle of autonomy or the principle of the greatest good for the greatest number. Interpreting ethics as a call to care challenges this approach in a different way by contending that the good is brought about by focusing on possibilities for fostering human well-being in the future. Thus, rather than seeking moral imperatives that require conformity based on a fixed system, moral imperative comes as an invitation to foster good by realizing future possibilities. The call to care comes as an invitation to share in a relationship that will foster future human well-being.

Nurses usually experience the call to care in everyday practice as particular visions that promise to foster the well-being of their patients. They seldom think of these visions as calls to care but merely as sound nursing care. The good to be fostered by nursing practice is so inherent in nursing care that it usually is not explicitly apparent to the caregiver. The call to care present in the practice often is explicitly recognized when unusual circumstances bring it to light. One aforementioned nurse recognized her calling when a mother profusely thanked her for saving her baby's life by giving mouth-to-mouth resuscitation. Although the nurse responded by saying that any competent nurse could and would have given mouth-to-mouth, her decision to remain in nursing indicates that she heard and responded to the call to care inherent in nursing practice.

In the past, interpreting health care as a response to calls to care often has been justified by a religious or philosophical foundation. This line of reasoning assumed that a person should be moral because human nature required it, the nature of the universe indicated it, or God demanded it. In our so-called post-modern age, such appeals to foundations no longer convince many people to respond to the call to care. Consequently, we will explore some calls to care that are nonfoundational. Unlike those who look for the one true calling, such as duty or compassion, we will treat many ways of calling. We will explore being called by good fortune, exemplars of care, the plight of others, professional competence and meaning, concrete relationships and situations, compassion, and the desire for authentic being.

1. Schweitzer: Good Fortune Obligates

Schweitzer has called many to care through his example of medical care for the natives of Lambaréné. Born to privilege and highly talented, he had become a well-known scholar when he decided that his good fortune obligated him to care for those less fortunate. His call was formulated as his second principle of ethics, which asserts that good fortune obligates. The second principle is far less known than his absolute first principle of reverence for life, according to Herbert Spiegelberg (1975). Schweitzer's second principle is a relative one. Those with the good fortune of being wealthy, healthy, well educated, skilled and talented are obligated to care for those who are less fortunate. From Schweitzer's principle it follows that those who can care for themselves should care for those who cannot. The young cannot care for themselves, and, therefore, parents and teachers should care for them by helping them learn to care for themselves. Likewise, the ill and debilitated cannot care for themselves, and, therefore, physicians and nurses should care for them by helping them to become capable of self-care. Care for the ill and debilitated is not limited to professionals, but should be a concern of all persons who have been spared illness and debilitation, according to Schweitzer.

> We who have lived through this ghastly time and who have suffered no or merely minor injury cannot get rid of a certain embarrassment at having fared so much better than they. It forces us to resolve to offer them a little more than some ordinary sympathy. They have the right to expect that again and again we meet them with reverence and with a kindly, understanding, patient readiness to help in everything—we who have been spared the heavy fate that has been laid upon them. (cited in Spiegelberg 1975, 232)

Schweitzer believed that those who have suffered pain and have recovered have a special call to care.

> Whoever has been delivered of pain must not think he is now free again and can return to life as if nothing has happened to him. Now that he knows

about pain and anxiety he must help to meet pain and anxiety as far as human power can and bring deliverance to others as he received deliverance. (cited in Spiegelberg 1975, 232)

Schweitzer's call for those who have suffered and have recovered to help those who are now suffering is a principle that is operative in modern health care in the many support groups in which those who become better or well help and comfort those suffering from similar illness and debilitation.

Spiegelberg contends that Schweitzer's second principle issues a call to care that evokes a new moral consciousness in those who have been blessed by good fortune.

> It is aimed at awakening and developing a moral sense that is usually dormant but that on special occasions can be brought to the surface. This is the way in which prophets have tried to shape the moral consciousness of mankind. In this sense Schweitzer too does not simply engage in moral philosophy but attempts to create a new moral consciousness, not by commandments or suggestion but by proclamation and "summons" leading a person to see by himself what he has not yet consciously "realized" in the full sense of this term, expressing seeing and doing at the same time. (Spiegelberg 1975, 232)

Such awakening requires more than a principle. It requires exemplars such as Schweitzer, who left the comfort and stimulation afforded a highly successful scholar in Europe to become a physician caring for the natives in Lambaréné.

Schweitzer's second principle is a more forceful call to care because he lived that principle. Disclosing the moral sense of health care concretely and giving a call to care are integrally related to each other. Exemplars in nursing ethics disclose the meaning of nursing care in ways that issue a call to care. For this reason, we have used many exemplars of good nursing care in this book.

2. Jesus: Called by the Plight of the Neighbor

Jesus used a parable to disclose the meaning of being a neighbor, to evoke compassion, and to issue a call to care. When a lawyer asked Jesus for an academic definition of neighbor, Jesus responded with the story of the Good Samaritan. The example of the Samaritan discloses the meaning of being a neighbor through a relationship involving nursing care.

> 29 But he, desiring to justify himself, said to Jesus, "And who is my neighbor?" 30 Jesus replied, "A man was going down from Jerusalem to Jericho, and fell among robbers, who stripped him and beat him, and departed, leaving him half dead. 31 Now by chance a priest was going

down that road; and when he saw him he passed by on the other side. [32] So likewise a Levite, when he came to the place and saw him, passed by on the other side. [33] But a Samaritan, as he journeyed, came to where he was; and when he saw him, he had compassion, [34] and went to him and bound up his wounds, pouring on oil and wine; then he set him on his own beast and brought him to an inn, and took care of him. [35] And the next day he took out two denarii and gave them to the innkeeper, saying, 'Take care of him; and whatever more you spend, I will repay you when I come back.' [36] Which of these three, do you think, proved neighbor to the man who fell among the robbers?" [37] He said, "The one who showed mercy on him." And Jesus said to him, "Go and do likewise." (Luke 10:29–37)

From the point of view of traditional philosophy, the dialogue between Jesus and the lawyer in verses 36 and 37 is disappointing. A philosopher would expect Jesus to give a definition of neighbor after giving such an excellent example of the meaning of neighbor. Instead, Jesus's question, "Which of these three do you think proved neighbor to the man who fell among the robbers?" subtly questions the intent of the lawyer. By his question, Jesus redirects the concern of the lawyer from an academic definition of neighbor to the concrete relationship of being a good neighbor. His concluding imperative, "Go and do likewise," indicates that knowing the meaning of being a neighbor issues a call to neighborly care.

The neighborly care exemplified by the Good Samaritan is nursing care. The Samaritan responds to the injured person by pouring oil and wine on the wounds, by bandaging them, by caring for him the remainder of the day, and by arranging for his recuperative care. But his call is to the nursing care of the common life. He is not a professional nurse specifically dedicated to caring for the injured with the specialized skill and knowledge that empowers that care.

Does being empowered as a nurse imply being available for care outside of health care institutions? The priest and Levite obviously did not believe that their special priestly abilities for care should be used with persons who were not part of their professional responsibilities. In contrast, the Samaritan felt called to care for a person who was probably a Jew, not a Samaritan. We do not know the injured man's religious tradition, because the Samaritan responded to him as a person who needed care, and not as someone for whom he had specific responsibility.

Having a similar sense of calling, a nurse responded to the call to care for three elderly neighbors when they were ill. She responded as a neighbor but as a specially empowered neighbor when health care was needed. Her response to their needs and their calling on her was predicated on her nursing ability and skill. She believed that nurses are called to care, not by their institutional employment, but by concern for the well-being of persons and by having a special empowerment to foster their well-being. The Good Samaritan is different from this nurse only in lacking special empowerment to engage in nursing care. Although this nurse had much greater proficiency in nursing care than the Samaritan, she was called to care by the plight of those who needed care in the same way that the Samaritan was called.

3. Pellegrino: The Call of Profession

Edmund Pellegrino (1985) interprets "profession" in a way that issues a call to care that encompasses the special abilities of physicians. He contends that the physician-patient relationship begins with a concrete request for care made by a person who is ill and seeks help. The physician accepts this request for help by the act of profession, in which the physician professes to be able to help the patient and to use his/her ability for the patient's well-being. This promise to use knowledge and skill for the well-being of the patient is, for Pellegrino, the essence of a profession. Thus, a profession has a moral foundation in which the professional professes to foster the well-being of those seeking help. For Pellegrino, health care professionals engage in health care by affirmative response to the call to care.

Is the call to care for nurses and physicians similar enough for a common calling to care? Pellegrino (1985) believes that both nursing and medicine share a common imperative to care for the ill and debilitated. In contrast, Sara Fry (1989) has contended that a caring relationship developed for a physician-patient relationship is not adequate for nurse-patient relationships. In making this contention, she referred to Pellegrino's interpretation of caring. There are four ways of caring in Pellegrino's interpretation of integral care. The first is compassion; the second is doing for others what they cannot do for themselves, because of illness and debilitation; the third is using knowledge and skill to care for the patient; the fourth is care involving the craft of health care (Pellegrino 1985). Regardless of differences in nursing and medical care, a caring relationship does call both nurse and physician into relationships with patients that involve compassion, direct care, knowledge and skill, and craft .

Pellegrino's description of the caring relationship, however, does seem more appropriate for physician-patient than for nurse-patient relationships. His description of caring assumes that health care giver and patient choose each other. In most nursing situations, this is rarely true for either nurse or patient. In addition, although Pellegrino points this out, physicians rarely do for patients what they can't do for themselves, such as bathing. Nurses, too, are less involved in such activities than they once were, although many recognize that personal care such as bathing affords an excellent opportunity for developing the nurse-patient relationship. Nevertheless, everyday nursing care often requires more intimate relationships between nurse and patient than the relationship between physician and patient. In addition,

Pellegrino focuses moral decision making on securing agreement between what is *medically* indicated and what is called for by the patient's view of the good life. What is medically indicated usually means prescribing a particular treatment, whereas nursing involves continuous ongoing care. Nurses often hear patients say, "It hurts to move," "I don't want to eat this food," "Don't make me get up," when restoring good health requires a patient to do all of these. Rather than prescribing, nurses engage in persuasive interaction that responds to patients' desires. Nursing care usually concerns ongoing care in which there is interaction between nurse and patient that calls for continual informing consent between what good nursing care requires and what the patient desires.

4. James: Concrete Calling

William James (1948), like Pellegrino, believed that we are called to be moral by our interaction with persons. James contended that we are called to moral action when others make concrete demands on us. He maintained "that without a claim actually made by some concrete person there can be no obligation, but that there is some obligation wherever there is a claim" (James 1948, 72). Thus for James, as for Pellegrino, the call to care is given concretely by specific persons.

The concrete call to care, for James, comes not only from specific persons but from the situations to which persons respond. He was wary of the "idealistic" version of calls to morality that were divorced from specific situations. He described such utopian divorcement from the world during a visit to a Chautauqua retreat. His feelings were elevated by the pleasant surroundings, wonderful lectures, good conversations, and excellent concerts. He described it as a middle-class heaven. Eventually he became uneasy because he felt divorced from the struggle and tension always present in the "real world."

As he journeyed from Lake Chautauqua, he passed through the steel mills of Buffalo and saw the laborers sweating and straining under conditions typical of most factory work in the latter nineteenth century in America. He then recalled how Tolstoy and others idealized the work of the common laborer. But when he examined the life of the common worker who merely struggled to exist, he found it wanting.

> The barrenness and ignobleness of the more usual laborer's life consist in the fact that it is moved by no such ideal inner springs. The backache, the long hours, the danger, are patiently endured—for what? To gain a quid of tobacco, a glass of beer, a cup of coffee, a meal, and a bed, and to begin again the next day and shirk as much as one can. (James 1958, 185)

Then he concluded that hard work and struggle alone did not make life worth living.

A life was worth living, for James, when moral vision of possible good called a person into a new way of being. This vision was not a general one addressed to everyone, but a concrete one. In living in specific situations with specific talents, a person would be called by a vision of possible good specifically addressed to the particular person at a certain time.

James's approach to ethics is evident in the relationship of Beverly and Midori. Midori's plight called Beverly into a caring relationship with her. The quality of that relationship gave Beverly a new vision of what it meant to be a good nurse, a vision that promised to inspire and guide her future nursing care. This interpretation of concrete calling is well suited for nursing ethics. Nurses are in situations in which the plight of the ill, the injustice of the situation, and the nature of their talents all call them to care in specific ways. James's contention that responding to moral calling makes life worth living is supported by our study of fulfillment in nursing (Bishop and Scudder 1990). In that study 39 of 40 nurses described their most fulfilling experience as a nurse as one in which they fulfilled their moral calling in specific situations.

5. Werner Marx: Called by Compassion

Werner Marx (1992) develops an ethics of compassion that is not founded in the Judeo-Christian or metaphysical traditions. Marx asserts that his "search for 'another' ethics is not motivated here by a position against the Judeo-Christian tradition" (Marx, 43). In fact, he believes that "nothing would be more desirable than a reassertion of the Judeo-Christian ethic" (43). But he believes that this foundation is no longer available to many persons.

Marx asks if we can be absolutely certain of anything in our age of relativity. His answer is that we are absolutely certain of our mortality. When I face my mortality, horror "dis-places me, in the true sense of this word, from all the familiar relations and habits pertaining to myself, to the things in my environment, and which above all ex-pels me from the everyday modes of being-with my fellow-men" (48–49). Marx contends that I, like all human beings, normally live in "the curious security of being of a nearly 'eternal kind of being'" (49) and comfortably relate to others through "interactions and communications in the common life-world" (49) as taken for granted, thing-like beings. In this taken-for-granted way of being, I am indifferent to others and to my own mortality. When the horror of my mortality shatters this indifference, I am open to the presence of others as fellow human beings. Isolated and forlorn, I need the presence of my brother or sister. Then, "I am not only able to *see* the other as my other . . . but also to *hear* his *call*" (52). Then "I hear and see the Other no longer in an indifferent attunement but in an attunement of extreme need. Thus, I hope to receive a 'sympathetic' response from him" (52).

When I see and hear my neighbors, I recognize them as sharing my fate. But does this shared fate make them my neighbors? For Marx, it does not necessarily make them neighbors but does free me from the "captivity of indifference" that prevents them from being my neighbors. When I am freed from indifference, I am freed to respond to the other's call to brotherhood or sisterhood. Responding to the other's call means that I treat him/her as an equal and with compassion.

Nurses care for patients who are being forced to face their own mortality in ways that can open them to the need for compassionate relations with others. People are often blinded to this need by regarding conventional ways of being with others as being compassionate and neighborly. For example, a person on hearing that his neighbor's wife is ill and in the hospital says, "I must go visit Joe; he is my neighbor." Neighbors conventionally call on each other in times of illness and misfortune. But when the neighbor hears that Joe's wife is dying, he responds, "Poor Joe, I must comfort him." This is the response of the neighbor who is shocked out of conventional ways by facing mortality. Nurses often respond to patients by relating to them in the conventional ways of the profession. They are often shocked out of treating this person as *the* patient in *this* professionally defined way by confronting their own mortality through their patient's mortality. Mutual facing of mortality often calls nurse and patient out of their shell of conventionality into authentic compassionate care for each other.

Facing mortality opens up the possibility of personal relationships, according to Marx, because people reach out for personal compassionate relationships. He believes that a person is always searching out others saying, "notice me, acknowledge me, relieve me from my loneliness, have compassion for me, love me. . . . He waits for neighborly love, he expects compassion" (60). When responded to with love and compassion, a person rejoices. "The fulfillment of the call of the person waiting for neighborly love releases joy in him, joy at having been heard, at having been listened to. . . . Joy is 'infectious' . . . . Joy . . . makes 'brothers' of all men wherever it dwells" (60).

For Marx, being with others as brothers and sisters makes life worth living and fills it with joy. The purpose of facing our mortality is to shatter the indifference that inhibits reaching out for brotherhood/sisterhood and compassion. Facing our mortality may shock us out of our everyday way of dealing with persons habitually. Marx's stress on the shock of facing our own mortality, however, seems to keep him from recognizing that his ethics of compassion is rooted in the human desire for compassion and brotherhood/sisterhood rather than in our common mortality.

Marx believes that we are communal beings who dwell in a life-world with language, institutions, and social relations. Without dwelling in the life-world, we could not be. Unfortunately, human beings, especially in our time, use the meanings and skills gained from participating in communal life to pursue their private interests rather than those of the community. Marx believes that this loss of community can be overcome by developing "the virtue of social sympathy against the background of the capacity for com-passion" (Marx, 70). Those who live in community experience the forms of love, sympathy, and acknowledgment in which human beings can dwell. Dwelling in these forms fosters the capacity for recognizing and measuring good and evil.

Communal practice of care often leads those who enter nursing merely as another job to discover its moral sense.

> I'll have to confess that I never did feel called into nursing. I feel like I fell into nursing. I think it had a lot to do with life experiences and situations, social contexts that I was embedded in at the time. I had the opportunity to have some work experiences in a hospital setting that oriented me to nursing. I had choices to make in college. I really didn't know what I wanted to do with my life. That was something I was familiar with. It was more comfortable and less threatening to enter into. As I learned more about nursing, as I got into the profession, I grew into it. I grew to love it, but I definitely did not feel called from the very beginning. (Lashley, Neal, Slunt, Berman, and Hultgren 1994, 7)

The above confession is given by Mary Lashley, one of the authors of a book entitled *Being Called to Care.* The call to care obviously did not initiate her entry into nursing but was given to her through being engaged in nursing practice with its inherent moral sense of care. Her call came from participating in an ongoing community whose ways of being called her to care.

Not only does Marx believe that our moral life is threatened by loss of communal life, he also believes it is endangered by the lack of unity in our life. He contends that it is no longer possible to construct or discover unity in *the* comprehensive system of philosophy sought by our rationalist tradition. Instead of seeking that kind of unity, he believes that we should rejoice in the richness of the plurality of meaning in our worlds and seek unity in the "force that permeates everything in the manner of a setting free" (85). This unifying force is the capacity for compassion (Marx, 127–140).

Nurses have sought unity through holistic interpretations in which the various fields of nursing are unified with each other and hopefully with the rest of health care. This so-called holistic approach, as we have argued elsewhere (Bishop and Scudder 1991, 78), is a Humpty Dumpty approach in that after health care is fractured by specialization, poor Humpty Dumpty is supposed to be put back together again. We have contended that the unity in health care comes from its moral sense—concern for the well-being of others. Marx calls us to seek unity through compassionate concern that fosters the well-being of patients. His call to unity speaks forcefully to nurses who believe that commitment to care for others is the source of the identity of nursing and of its unity.

6. Taylor: The Call to Authenticity

Whereas Marx develops an ethics of compassion that issues a call to care, Charles Taylor (1991) gives a philosophical interpretation of the ethics of authenticity that can call nurses to care. The call to care implicit in an ethics of authenticity is often missed because, as Taylor points out, neither the critics nor the defenders of authenticity do justice to its ethical import. The defenders and critics both place authenticity within an ethical relativism that makes choice itself focal. Taylor points out that choice is insignificant without some means of determining that one choice is better than another. He contends that authenticity is morally significant when it commits persons to choose to pursue the best, given their potential and situation in the world.

> The moral ideal behind self-fulfillment is that of being true to oneself, in a specifically modern understanding of that term. . . . What do I mean by moral ideal? I mean a picture of what a better or higher mode of life would be, where "better" and "higher" are defined not in terms of what we happen to desire or need, but offer a standard of what we ought to desire. (Taylor 1991, 15–16).

This interpretation of authenticity can enlighten Noddings's ethical caring. In her interpretation of caring, when I do not care naturally, I should care because I want to be a caring person. Translated into nursing, this would mean that I care for clients even when I do not naturally care for them, because I recognize caring as the way I ought to be. In so doing, I would be authentic in that I would be following the vision of what I "ought to desire," namely being in a caring relationship that fosters the well-being of others. Thus, a nurse who cares for patients because she/he wants to become a caring person would be an authentic nurse, just as would be a nurse who cared out of natural caring, because both are being led by what they ought to desire—being in a caring relationship that fosters the well-being of their patients.

Taylor's interpretation of the moral sense of authenticity is valuable to nurses who wish to foster authenticity in patients by giving them authentic care. We have previously discussed authentic care in the following way.

> Heidegger (1962) . . . contrasts two ways of caring for others. In the first way, a person will *"leap in"* for another and "take over for the other." This form of care can readily foster domination and dependency when the caregiver "leaps in and takes away 'care.'" We will call this dependent care because it fosters dependency on others. In contrast to dependent care, authentic care (so named by Heidegger) occurs when the caregiver will *"leap ahead* of him [ihm vorausspringt] in his existentiell (sic) potentiality-for-Being, not in order to take away his 'care' but rather to give it back to him authentically" (158–159). Thus, in authentic care the other is helped to care for his or her own being. (Bishop and Scudder 1991, 56)

Nurses who have been in practice for a long time will recognize that much of the care given earlier in this century was dependent care. Increasingly nurses have become aware of the value of authentic care that frees patients to direct their own being. Such care requires greater stress on patient education and on encouraging clients to take responsibility for their health care. Taylor's moral sense of authenticity would require nurses to move a step further by helping persons to discover possibilities for becoming their best selves during and after illness and treatment.

Sally Gadow's (1980) contention that nurses ought to be existential advocates calls for nurses to help patients become more authentic by the way they care for them. By existential advocacy, she means helping patients discover the meaning of illness and treatment for their lives, and encouraging and assisting them in following that meaning. The nurse as existential advocate cannot merely help patients choose what they want—for example, the drug user who wants to be as "high" as possible while in the hospital. The existential advocate is there to help patients recognize and realize their best selves, given their situation.

The stress in medical ethics on decisions concerning to-treat or not-to-treat often obscures the moral imperative to assist patients in discovering and pursuing their best selves in a given health care situation. This is evident in the case that we discussed in the first chapter, in which a patient with mania refused to take Lithium because he wanted to remain high. Both the ethicist and the physicians were so focused on the issue of whether to-treat or not-to-treat that they failed to discuss with the patient the moral issues involved in his decision not to take Lithium. Further, they seemed not to recognize the moral imperative to help the patient discover and realize his best self. Ethical considerations could have led this patient to consider what would be best for his life rather than merely what would foster his pleasure. Such considerations make ethics an integral aspect of therapy itself, since they involve helping patients discover and choose what they ought to desire for future well-being rather than what they presently desire. For example, an elderly person with a broken hip desires to avoid pain, but her nurse encourages her to face the pain in order to be able to walk again and thus become a more independent person.

That moral considerations could be an essential ingredient in therapy itself is often obscured by the tendency to interpret nursing as an applied or behavioral science. This interpretation often denies that persons are capable of desiring and choosing to pursue future possible good in given situations— an assumption that underlies Taylor's interpretation of authenticity. Social scientists do this, according to Taylor, by attributing behavior to non-moral factors, such as the desire for survival, power, control, or wealth, in an attempt to give explanations that are "hard" and "scientific" (Taylor 1991, 20). Applying this stance in nursing, as we have argued in our previous books, has blinded nurses to the moral sense inherent in its practice. Consequently, we believe, with Taylor, that retrieval of "this ideal can help us restore our practice" (23).

An ethics of authenticity makes its claim on me in a way uniquely appropriate to my way of being and my situation, according to Taylor. This unique calling means that my identity cannot be "socially derived but must be inwardly generated" (47). Forming my identity requires inward generation called forth by the world.

> I alone experience myself as a subject but I experience myself in a world that makes demands on me and in interaction with others that fosters self-understanding. Inward generation of self-definition is initiated by a call from the world. . . . Only if I exist in a world in which history, or the demands of nature, or the needs of my fellow human beings, or the duties of citizenship, or the call of God, or something else of this order *matters* crucially, can I define an identity for myself that is not trivial. Authenticity is not the enemy of demands that emanate from beyond the self; it supposes such demands. (Taylor 1991, 40–41)

The call to moral commitment that emanates from beyond the self is often given by working with others through "horizons of significance" (Taylor, 38). In nursing, these horizons of significance constitute the meanings that orient nursing practice. A nurse does not define herself/himself out of an inward generation divorced from practice, but through the meanings embedded in practice. The essential meaning of practice is a moral sense— caring for the well-being of others.

Novice nurses who have a strong sense of being called to care often have difficulty relating this call to the practice of nursing. We found in our study of fulfillment in nursing that nursing students need to learn how the call to care is carried out in practice. The forty senior nursing students we compared with forty practicing nurses felt most fulfilled when care referred to personal relationships. But these relationships, unlike those of the experienced nurses, tended to be divorced from the practice of caring for patients in clinical situations. For example, one nursing student, who regarded nursing as "being enabled to care empathetically for those less fortunate," described her most fulfilling nursing experience as being at the beck and call of her patient to do favors that had marginal relationship to nursing practice. In contrast, in the descriptions of care for patients by experienced nurses, the personal and moral were so often disclosed in professional and technical language that Jack often needed a translation into lay terms by Anne in order for him to grasp the moral and personal significance of their care. Regardless of how technical the descriptions of the care that brought these nurses fulfillment, they were all examples of fulfilling the moral sense of nursing in ways that were responses to the call to care given in actual practice.

If our study accurately depicts the prevalence of the moral sense in nursing, why are the moral sense and the call to care so neglected? Nurses are socialized to describe their nursing experiences in the technical and professional language of nursing in ways that obscure the moral sense and the sense of being called to care. In nursing literature and education, the term "professional" is often substituted for the moral imperative. When nurses do not practice as they ought to practice, they usually are not charged with being immoral but with being unprofessional. For example, when nurses abandon a patient needing round-the-clock supervision, in order to gossip with colleagues in the lounge, they are usually charged with being unprofessional rather than with being immoral. The charge of immorality is usually reserved for cases that are included under such terms as "moral turpitude." Charges of moral turpitude are usually concerned with unacceptable conduct that seldom directly affects patient care.

Nurses are charged with being unprofessional when they deviate from professionally established criteria. This way of thinking comes from interpreting nursing as a profession in the sociological rather than the moral sense. The sociological definition of profession includes having a body of knowledge, educational standards, criteria for judging competent performance, and a code of ethics. One motivating factor in developing the code of ethics for nursing has been to establish nursing as a profession. This probably accounts for the failure of the code to give significant direction to nursing practice, even when the code sets sound standards for what nursing ought to be.

One problem with the sociological definition of profession is that it is arrived at by consensus. Definition by consensus eliminates the moral sense. Morality cannot be determined by consensus without losing the normative sense that is essential to morality. Pellegrino (1985) makes this clear in his moral interpretation of profession. He argues that contending that the American Medical Association (AMA) Code of Ethics is morally binding because it has been proclaimed by the leadership of the AMA as the consensus of the medical profession puts the cart before the horse. Medicine is a profession if, and only if, it is true to what it professes, namely, to use medical skill and knowledge to foster the well-being of the patient. A profession receives its special privileges from living up to its moral profession. Therefore, the profession does not establish the moral sense. The moral sense constitutes the profession.

Another way in which the moral sense of nursing is obscured is by viewing nursing as a morally neutral technological activity. Technology, for Taylor, is a concrete form of the instrumental reason that has become the dominant way of thinking in our society. He points out that both critics of instrumental reasoning and its uncritical advocates usually put it in a framework of dominance and control.

> We are free when we can remake the conditions of our own existence, when we can dominate the things that dominate us. Obviously this ideal helps to lend even greater importance to technological control over our world; it helps to enframe instrumental reason in a project of domination, rather than serving to limit it in the name of other ends. (Taylor 1991, 101)

Unfortunately, neither critics nor advocates seek another context for technology other than domination.

The uncritical advocates of instrumental reason believe that it is *the* way to solve all of our problems. They situate problems so that the technical sense, rather than moral sense, has priority. Instrumental reason "offers an ideal picture of a human thinking that has disengaged from its messy embedding in our bodily constitution, our dialogical situation, our emotions, and our traditional life forms in order to be pure, self-verifying rationality" (Taylor 1991, 101–102).

When instrumental reasoning was initiated into the West by Francis Bacon, according to Taylor, Bacon proposed "a model of science whose criterion of truth would be instrumental efficacy. You have discovered something when you can intervene to change things" (Taylor, 104). Modern science, including medical science, has followed Bacon in this respect. However, modern science has forgotten that the thrust behind Baconian science "was not only epistemological but also moral" (104). Bacon proposed using science to intervene in nature in order to foster human well-being.

Taylor believes that both the naive critics and supporters of instrumental reason have lost sight of the beneficent intent that fostered instrumental reason's rise to prominence.

> We can see what this kind of reflection involves if we look at one important example, from the field of medical care. Under (a), we note that the ideal of disengaged reason must be considered precisely as an ideal and not as a picture of human agency as it really is. We are embodied agents, living in dialogical conditions, inhabiting time in a specifically human way, that is, making sense of our lives as a story that connects the past from which we have come to our future projects. That means (b) that if we are properly

to treat a human being, we have to respect this embodied, dialogical, temporal nature. Runaway extensions of instrumental reason, such as the medical practice that forgets the patient as a person, that takes no account of how the treatment relates to his or her story and thus of the determinants of hope and despair, that neglects the essential rapport between cure-giver and patient—all these have to be resisted in the name of the moral background in benevolence that justifies these applications of instrumental reason themselves. If we come to understand why technology is important here in the first place, then it will of itself be limited and enframed by an ethic of caring. (Taylor 1991, 105–106)

Nurses who limit technology to a context of dominance can learn much from Taylor's critique. Nurses who oppose technology as a form of dominance usually restrict moral considerations of nursing to personal relationships. Advocates of technology who place it in the context of dominating nature usually regard nursing primarily as intervention. Taylor shows that technology belongs in a context other than dominance. He contends that we need to understand technology "in the moral frame of the ethic of practical benevolence, which is also one of the sources in our culture from which instrumental reason has acquired its salient importance for us" (106).

Taylor's treatment of technology reveals the method he uses throughout his book *The Ethics of Authenticity* (1991). He attempts to "identify and articulate the higher ideal behind . . . practices, and then criticize these practices from the standpoint of their own motivating ideal" (72). Instead of dismissing or endorsing a practice, Taylor contends that we ought to make evident what it means in terms of its motivating ideal and then point out what being true to that ideal really involves. Taylor's method, when applied to the purpose of this book, would require us to recover the essential and authentic meaning of nursing practice and then to test and judge the worth of nursing practice by the extent to which it fulfills its moral sense. We have, without explicitly following Taylor's approach, used a similar approach in our ongoing attempt to develop a philosophy of nursing. We have claimed that nursing is the practice of caring and that it has the inherent moral sense of fostering the well-being of others. This means that nursing ethics would primarily concern how well the moral sense of nursing is being fulfilled by individual nurses and by the nursing profession. Further, since the worth of nursing itself would be judged by how it fulfills its moral sense, moral concerns would not be peripheral or add-on concerns to nursing's professional and technical activities, but would form the very heart of nursing practice itself.

Nurses who practice in highly technical situations are no less called to care than those whose practice involves more hands-on and personal care. They are called to care technically. But if the call to technical efficiency is their primary calling, they are technicians rather than nurses. This does not mean that technical efficiency is unimportant or that nurses should not feel pride and fulfillment from technical competency. It does mean that a nurse's call to be technical must be enframed in an ethics of care. The ultimate call for nurses is the call to care. The call to care, unlike the contingent call of technical competence, is itself a moral calling.

The Integral Calling of Compassion and Authenticity

If moral calling is to act out of compassion to care for the well-being of clients, can nurses be expected to respond authentically to this calling? It would make no sense to say that nurses ought to be compassionate, in the same way that we say nurses should act to foster the well-being of patients. Being compassionate is not something that human beings can achieve by an act of will. It is possible to be open to compassion, to situate yourself so that compassion is likely to be evoked, and to follow the call of compassion. In the parable of the Good Samaritan, the priest and the Levite who passed by on the other side, in contrast to the Samaritan, were not open to the calling and direction of compassion. The ethical question with regard to compassion, rather than being "Ought I be compassionate?" should be "Ought I be open to compassion, to give myself to it, and to act out of it?" Acting compassionately usually finds itself in tension with other ways of being, such as self-serving, detached objective observation, seeking the truth, comfort-seeking, cowardly retreat, or desiring the approval of others. Thus, an ethics of compassion concerns being open to the call of compassion and being willing to respond to that call by fostering the well-being of the person whose situation initially evoked the compassion. The Good Samaritan is morally commendable not because he felt compassion but because he was open to compassion and allowed it to foster good nursing care for the injured person. The Good Samaritan is authentic in that his nursing care followed naturally from his compassion, and he chose to act out of that compassion.

What of nurses who do not feel compassion but feel called to care? They can, according to Noddings, be called to care out of the desire to be a caring person by entering a caring relationship with those who need care. I am moral when I choose to be in that caring way that fosters the well-being of others. This, according to Taylor, would make me authentic, in that I am choosing to follow what I ought to desire—being in caring relationships with those who need my care. Thus, I can be an authentic person by choosing to follow compassion or by choosing what I ought to desire—to be a caring person.

In nursing when I choose to follow compassion authentically, I naturally foster the well-being of my clients. When compassion is not present, I am called to care by my desire to be a caring nurse and by the caring way of being evoked by nursing practice. Choosing to be a caring nurse requires me to engage in a caring relationship focused on fostering the patient's well-being. The moral sense of nursing practice invites me to enter authentically into caring relationships with my clients and gives me ways of caring for their well-being. In authentic care we are called to care out of a desire to be caring persons and to be excellent practitioners who care for the well-being of clients. In compassionate care, we are called directly to care for their well-being. When the call to care is a call to act out of compassion, out of the desire to be a caring nurse, and out of authentic participation in caring practice, three powerful sources of morality come together to foster compassionate authentic care for those whose plight calls for care.

Study Questions

1. In what ways does the relationship of Beverly and Midori call nurses to care? What other ways can you think of?
2. Why does Chinn believe that being called to care is the appropriate way to speak of becoming a caring person?
3. Some critics of contemporary morality argue that the only way to restore the moral fiber of our people is to return to the philosophical and religious foundations that once called people to care. Others argue that such contentions merely state the problem rather than offer the solution to our lack of moral conviction. The problem is that we no longer accept and respond to traditional moral foundations. Which position do you agree with? Why?
4. Discuss the meaning of Schweitzer's contention that good fortune obligates. Why do Anne and Jack believe that exemplars such as Schweitzer's medical care are needed in ethics?
5. How is the call to care given to the Good Samaritan different from that of a nurse? How is it similar?
6. What are the four ways of caring in Pellegrino's interpretation of integral care? Do you agree with Fry's contention that Pellegrino's caring relationship is inadequate for nursing? Why or why not?
7. How does James's "concrete calling" call nurses to care? Give an example of a concrete call to care that you have experienced.
8. Why does Marx contend that facing our mortality opens us to the possibility of compassionate and neighborly relationships with others? What implications does his contention have for nursing care?

9. Do you think that Marx's view on unity can help nursing achieve unity in our time of specialization and cultural pluralism? Why or why not?

10. How is Taylor's interpretation of authenticity different from the views of both the critics and defenders of authenticity?

11. Why does Taylor reject choosing what we want or need as the meaning of authenticity? Why does he reject placing authenticity in a context of dominance? Give examples of claims to being authentic in nursing that Taylor would reject and examples that he would favor.

12. In what way does Taylor's interpretation of authenticity contribute to Noddings's conception of ethical caring?

13. How can technical and professional interpretations of nursing obscure its moral sense? How is it possible for nurses to be professionally and technically competent and still recognize nursing's moral sense?

14. How can Marx's interpretation of compassion and Taylor's interpretation of authenticity help unite Noddings's natural caring and ethical caring into a call to compassionate authentic care?

References

Bishop, Anne H., and John R. Scudder, Jr. (1990). *The Practical, Moral, and Personal Sense of Nursing: A Phenomenological Philosophy of Practice.* Albany, N.Y. : State University of New York Press.

Bishop, Anne H., and John R. Scudder, Jr. (1991). *Nursing: The Practice of Caring.* New York: The National League for Nursing Press.

Chinn, Peggy. (1994). Foreword to *Being Called to Care* by Mary Ellen Lashley, Maggie T. Neal, Emily Todd Slunt, Louise M. Berman, and Francine H. Hultgren. Albany, N.Y.: State University of New York Press.

Dyck, Beverly. (1989). The Paper Crane. *American Journal of Nursing* 89:824–825.

Fry, Sara T. (1989). Toward a Theory of Nursing Ethics. *Advances in Nursing Science* 11(4): 9–22.

Gadow, Sally. (1980). Existential Advocacy: Philosophical Foundation of Nursing. In *Nursing: Images and Ideals: Opening Dialogue with the Humanities,* eds. S. F. Spicker and Sally Gadow. New York: Springer.

Heidegger, Martin. (1962). *Being and Time.* trans. J. Macquarrie and E. Robinson. New York: Harper and Row.

Holy Bible, Revised Standard Version.

James, William. (1948). The Moral Philosopher and the Moral Life. In *Essays in Pragmatism,* ed. A. Castell. New York: Hafner Press.

James, William. (1958). *Talks to Teachers on Psychology: And to Students on Some of Life's Ideals.* New York: W. W. Norton.

Lashley, Mary Ellen, Maggie T. Neal, Emily Todd Slunt, Louise M. Berman, and Francine H. Hultgren. (1994). *Being Called to Care.* Albany, N.Y.: State University of New York Press.

Marx, Werner. (1992). *Toward a Phenomenological Ethics: Ethos and the Life-World.* Albany, N.Y.: State University of New York Press.

Pellegrino, Edmund. (1985). The Caring Ethic. In *Caring, Curing, Coping: Nurse, Physician, Patient Relationships,* eds. Anne H. Bishop and John R. Scudder, Jr., 8–30. University, Ala.: University of Alabama Press.

Spiegelberg, Herbert. (1975). Good Fortune Obligates: Albert Schweitzer's Second Ethical Principle. *Ethics* 86:227–234.

Taylor, Charles. (1991). *The Ethics of Authenticity.* Cambridge, Mass.: Harvard University Press.

5

Therapeutic Ethics

Treating ethics as a call to care may seem odd to those who regard nursing ethics as applied ethics. The concept of therapeutic ethics may sound even stranger. But it should make sense to advocates of an ethics of practice, because the moral sense of fostering the well-being of clients is common to both therapy and practice.

Health care ethics can be applied ethics or an ethics of practice. In applied ethics, the traditional ways for making ethical decisions, practiced by philosophers, are applied to actual medical and nursing cases. In contrast, an ethics of practice begins with the moral sense of health care and interprets ethics as consideration of how appropriately and how well the moral sense of health care is being fulfilled. What is at issue in the two approaches is not the extent to which actual cases or traditional philosophical ethics are involved in ethical considerations, but the fundamental orientation of ethics. For example, Robert Veatch and Sara Fry contend "that one cannot approach any ethics, especially nursing ethics, in the abstract" (Veatch and Fry 1987, 1). Although they focus their book on cases, they contend that nursing ethics is a branch of biomedical ethics, which in turn is a branch of philosophical ethics. The approach to the cases in their book is an applied approach to ethics. In contrast, those who orient health care ethics in the moral sense of health care generally regard health care ethics as clinical, rather than applied, ethics. Most books on nursing ethics follow the applied ethics approach. This book takes the other approach.

As far as we know, no one who has written a nursing ethics book has taken the clinical approach. Richard Zaner (1988) has developed clinical ethics in medicine in a way that lends itself to nursing ethics. We have, through the years, worked closely with Zaner and have frequently discussed with him the implications of his clinical ethics for nursing ethics. In this chapter, we will begin with Zaner's clinical ethics but then will show that his medical ethics moves from clinical ethics, as set forth in his book *Ethics and the Clinical Encounter* (1988), toward therapeutic ethics in his latest book, *Troubled Voices* (1993). Our purpose in this reinterpretation is not to give an adequate interpretation of Zaner's ethics but to gain insight and understanding that will contribute to developing an ethics of practice appropriate for nursing.

Zaner, in developing his clinical ethics, rejects the assumption of most traditional ethics that a moral person is primarily an autonomous, detached, rational decision maker. This approach, he contends, is based on two questionable assumptions. First, the self is self-contained, insulated from others, and has only its own thoughts and feelings. Second, other persons are not experienced directly but are inferred from sensory experiences of the other's body (Zaner 1988). Zaner rejects both assumptions. He contends that human beings, rather than being isolated and insulated, are beings who develop by mutuality and shared relationships. The moral life, rather than being an autonomous, rational application of abstract principles, is essentially mutual and communal. Whereas Zaner has shown how the detached, rational, autonomous approach does not make sense in medical practice, we have shown in previous work that it does not make sense in nursing practice.

> Nurses know that the above assumptions are unsound from their own experience. If the self is autonomous, in that it is closed in on itself, and therefore unable to grasp another person's meaning directly, nursing as practiced would be impossible. If a nurse can only infer meaning from a person's bodily movement rather than grasp the meaning from the body's expressiveness, nursing practice would certainly have to be altered. Imagine trying to turn a patient on a bed with efficiency and care to avoid unnecessary suffering if each grimace, body tension, grunt and moan, was to be taken as a sign from which to infer what was going on inside the body and then be correlated to the appropriate technique inferred from each sign. Instead, most nurses immediately recognize what the patient's bodily expressions mean and move him appropriately drawing on long years of practical experience. (Bishop and Scudder 1990, 125–126).

Showing that some traditional ways of thinking in ethics do not suit clinical situations does not tell us what an appropriate ethics for clinical situations would be. Zaner contends that such an ethics would have to meet three requirements.

Zaner's Requirements for a Clinical Ethics

1. The work of ethics requires strict focus on the specific situational definition of each involved person.
2. Moral issues are presented solely within the contexts of their actual occurrence.
3. The situational participants are the principal resources for the resolution of the moral issues presented.

From *Ethics and the Clinical Encounter* by Richard Zaner. Copyright 1988. Englewood Cliffs, NJ: Prentice Hall. pp. 243, 244, 246.

From these three requirements, Zaner develops a clinical ethics that works on behalf of all participants in the situation, including those who receive care—patients, families, friends—and the caregivers—physicians, nurses and others—and also the caregiving institution and its civic and social supporters. Such an ethics requires good communication between the participants, especially skill in listening to clients and using language that is understandable by them. Good communication requires a skilled probing to determine what is bothering those involved and how they understand their situation. The goal of communication is to help people make their own decisions concerning care and treatment, based upon their own beliefs and values.

Clinical ethics, for Zaner, is primarily concerned with enablement rather than with providing authoritative solutions to moral problems. Those involved in health care situations are the resources necessary to enable all involved to reach satisfactory solutions and adequate regimens of care. They are the ones who will have to live with the consequences of their decisions and actions. For Zaner, enablement means "that communicative process whereby situational participants are provided with the understanding, the means, opportunities, power, or authority, already intrinsic to their situation, to effect change by their decisions" (Zaner 1988, 248).

Zaner places health care ethics within the context of the clinical situation rather than within the context of traditional philosophical ethics. Those of us who believe that health care ethics should begin with the inherent moral sense of practice favor this move. However, labeling an ethics by the context in which it is placed may be questionable. For example, Joseph Fletcher took the name of his situational ethics from its situational context rather than from its motivating force, namely love. Fletcher's ethics could have been more appropriately labeled a love ethics—a love ethics that differentiated itself from other love ethics by taking seriously its situational context. Zaner's clinical ethics may also suffer from being defined by the situation in which it is placed. We believe that it should be termed a therapeutic ethics that is appropriately placed in a clinical context.

We came to the conclusion that Zaner's ethics is a therapeutic ethics by reading and interpreting his descriptions of his practice as an ethicist in his book *Troubled Voices: Stories of Ethics and Illness* (1993). From interpreting Zaner's examples of his work as an ethicist, we concluded that not only could Zaner's ethics be articulated as a therapeutic ethics but so could nursing ethics.

The case that disclosed to us that nursing ethics could be a therapeutic ethics was recommended to us by Zaner as one that spoke forcefully to nursing ethics.

Recently I received a call from a physician who wanted me to stop by to see a young man who had been hospitalized and was refusing hemodialysis. Refusal of treatment meant death. The patient was in his late twenties, and he had been hospitalized numerous times the previous summer for all manner of problems and was apparently just fed up with everything. . . .

He had been born with spina bifida, making him paraplegic and hydrocephalic, and had a surgically implanted shunt that took the cerebral-spinal fluid from his brain to his abdomen. . . .

That summer he had began [sic] to suffer from severe diarrhea, dehydration, infections, and a malfunctioning bladder and was repeatedly hospitalized. As if all that were not enough, his kidneys had begun to fail and he had become anemic. Now, hospitalized again, he staunchly refused to have dialysis even though it held the promise of at least some benefit, even a return to home and possibly the job he had held for some years. His physician, thinking that the young man was experiencing depression, prescribed an antidepressant hoping that he might, in a less distressed state, change his mind. . . .

But despite the antidepressant, he continued to refuse dialysis. Within a few days, the poisons inevitably built up and dialysis was seriously needed. His mother was terrified. His physician had gone out of town for the weekend and the resident and nurses seemed at loggerheads with this patient's persistent refusal.

In the press of circumstances, the physician covering for the attending decided to have a psychiatrist assess his competence. Surely, it was thought, no one in his right mind would refuse treatments that promised relief and return to normalcy. Unsurprisingly, by that time the psychiatrist found him "temporarily incompetent," and his "decision against dialysis" was taken to be a function of depression and failing thought processes, said to be caused by the build-up of poisons in his bloodstream. Armed with that, the covering physician was able to place the catheter and take him off to be dialyzed.

When the attending returned he was quite concerned—furious is probably more accurate. Not only had his patient been dialyzed despite refusing it the previous week, but here the young man was alert once again—the dialysis had, after all, done its thing—and very disturbed at being forced to have dialysis. In fact, he continued his adamant refusal of any further sessions with the dialysis machine. Both the attending and his mother were in a bind: both wanted to respect what they considered to be the young man's competently expressed refusal though knowing that dialysis was actually beneficial. But he said that he had had enough; in fact a lifetime of enough. . . .

I came back to see Tom and his mother. . . . We moved directly to the issues at hand. Did he understand the implications of his refusal of dialysis? In a way, he did; but as we talked it seemed to me that he hadn't thought it out at all well. He was in fact behaving rather differently than one would expect when meeting someone firmly refusing potentially life-saving treatment. It's not that he was calmly accepting. He had not in fact discussed the matter with his mother; he had not really even thought about it much for himself. He had not signed any advanced directive; the idea hadn't even occurred to him. And his mother had not raised the issue with him of the advanced directive or the clear consequence of his refusal. The thought that he would die without dialysis had, so to speak, sort of sidled past his awareness now and then, but he had not confronted matters squarely. . . .

Trying to learn more about Tom personally, I asked him about his job, one which he obviously enjoyed and in which he took some pride. It was an office-type position with a state agency, and it had given him a good deal of independence. Before he became so sick some months ago, he had even started to think he could get his own apartment and begin to live on his own. *That*, it seemed to me, was what was really on his mind. The numerous illnesses and hospitalizations had eventually required him to quit his job, which more than anything else seemed the source of his depression. Like all of us at one time or another, he had it all "figured out": on dialysis he would not be able to hold a job, much less go back to the one he really liked—*ergo*, life ain't worth it, so let's just give up. Being "normal," working and living independently, had become an insurmountable goal when viewed from his perspective.

He continued talking and I listened. A few months ago, he said, almost as an afterthought, he had been told by his supervisor that his job would be waiting for him when he was able to return. As soon as he said this he noticeably perked up; his talk became more lively, his gestures more animated.

"That's right," his mother quickly affirmed, "Mrs. Y did say you could have your job back when you're able."

"But how can I work," Tom's tremulous words seemed at once hopeful and wary, "when I've got to be on that damned machine so much?"

His mother and I vied with each other to get the thing said: work was indeed possible. Hadn't he discussed this with his doctor? He wasn't sure. Perhaps he had been so wrapped up in grief and a deep sense of loss that he hadn't heard. Or perhaps none of his doctors had thought to mention it, or if any of them had, Tom hadn't understood. In any event, it was clear that the way things appeared had changed dramatically for him. I suggested that he really needed to find out much more about dialysis and to call up his supervisor to check with her about returning to work. . . . It was perfectly obvious that he did not want to refuse dialysis and that he desperately wanted to get out of the hospital and back to work. . . .

The last time I visited Tom he was on the dialysis machine. He told me that his boss had told him that he could have his old job back. He was very upbeat, joshing about the machine, joking with his nurse, and offering to come to one of my classes and talk about himself. (Zaner 1993, 47–55)

From *Troubled Voices: Stories of Ethics and Illness* by Richard Zaner. Copyright 1993 by Richard M. Zaner, Jr. Cleveland, Ohio: Pilgrim Press. Used with permission.

In reconsidering this clinical encounter, Zaner was haunted by a series of questions. "When Tom first expressed his refusal to undergo dialysis, shouldn't that have had priority? Did his decline into renal psychosis change the competency with which he chose that condition? The decline, after all, was exactly what one would expect to occur. Within a day or so, he would have lapsed into an irreversible coma and then died. And wasn't this just what he had chosen?" (Zaner 1993, 54) Had it not been for a fortuitous lack of communication between two physicians, his decision would have been honored, his rights respected, and he would have died.

Tom, however, had chosen to forego treatment without adequate knowledge of how dialysis would affect his life, especially his job and his desire to be more independent. Those who discussed this matter with Tom did so in the context of to-treat or not-to-treat and of Tom's *right* to deny treatment if competent. But why had no one inquired about the reason for his despondency and feeling of hopelessness? Zaner, called in as an ethicist, did inquire, but why hadn't Tom's physician or nurse done so? Why had they limited their concern to whether or not to give the dialysis that would make his continued living possible? Why had they not, as Zaner did, helped Tom discover what would make his life meaningful enough to endure dialysis? Tom knew well the suffering and limitations of a life dependent on medicine and on others. As he said, "He had had a lifetime of enough!" Therefore, his refusal of dialysis did not result from being of unsound mind, but from not knowing his own mind. He needed to discover what would make a dialysis-dependent life worth living. Zaner, by entering his life-world, helped him to make the discovery that restored him to mental health, physical health, and the moral good for his life.

Ethics is therapeutic for Zaner because of the way he interprets both ethics and therapy. This is evident in his comments concerning Tom. "We sense how deeply Tom felt torn away from what he had most wanted to be, compellingly pulled to keep alive his hope for independence even while he thought it was lost, as dead as he thought he now wanted to be. But it was not death, but a particular way of being alive that he most wanted" (Zaner 1993, 142). For Zaner, therapy is not limited to bodily functions fostered by chemical and surgical interventions but concerns the well-being of the whole person considered in light of that person's medical situation. For Zaner, ill persons like Tom find themselves faced "with a basic challenge to their sense of self. What and who we are, what we hope to be and become, even whether we will continue to be at all, is in one way or another at stake in these circumstances. This poses basic moral questions" (Zaner 1993, 137). Thus, moral issues are posed, for Zaner, by facing the problem of our own being and becoming, in light of illness or debilitation and possible treatments to alleviate them. An ethicist helps persons place their illness, debilitation, and treatment within the context of patients' being and becoming as expressed in their beliefs and values.

People usually do not reflect on their basic beliefs and values in day to day living. Illness, debilitation, and treatment call forth such reflection. Working with an ethicist becomes the occasion for such difficult, disquieting, and insightful reflection (Zaner 1993, 147). Zaner believes that the ethicist's job is to serve as the philosophical therapist rather than as an expert who instructs patients on moral decision making, using traditional ethical procedures and norms. By exploring possible actions in light of beliefs and values in a clinical context, Zaner hopes to help people come to their own decisions. These decisions often come about with sudden clarity.

When the dialysis patient, Tom, for instance, began talking about his job and his hopes of getting an apartment, a veritable transformation took place in his gestures and words. I could almost see a light bulb go on. He was suddenly enlivened, talking about how he would get back to work, get an apartment. Yet only a moment before, he had been muted, his gestures slow and heavy, his voice and words softened by sadness, grief, loss. (Zaner 1993, 149)

Zaner believes that clinical ethics helps people to come to "Ah-ha!" experiences that bring into focus how what is important in their lives relates to their health care.

For Zaner, an ethicist creates a caring therapeutic relationship in which decisions are made in the context of being cared for and being treated with respect. These therapeutic relationships are created by affiliation and compassion. In a relationship of affiliation, the therapist reaches out to others in order to see their situation from their points of view. In a relationship of compassion, the therapist enters into a relationship of "feeling-with-others" (Zaner 1993, 146).

For Zaner, ethics in health care is therapeutic. The moral sense of health care is not only evident in his therapeutic ethics but is constitutive of it. He affirms the integral relation between ethics and health care practice that often is obscured by viewing ethics as an adjunct activity to medical and nursing therapy. Those who hold the adjunct view believe that ethics is needed to resolve moral problems that are tangential to therapy. Rather than arguing directly for the integral relationship between ethics and therapy, Zaner discloses that ethics is therapeutic by interpreting well-chosen examples. The example we considered illustrates how his practice and his interpretation of his practice disclose the therapeutic nature of ethics. His description discloses the therapeutic meaning of health care ethics and at the same time evokes in his readers a moral concern for the ill. Rather than the traditional opposition between the detachment of traditional ethics and the caring presence of therapy, Zaner's therapy expresses his concern for the well-being of the ill and how ethicists can foster that well-being. His therapy is directed at fostering the patient's well-being. He describes that therapy and articulates its meaning in a way that enhances the ethicist's ability and commitment to foster the well-being of the patient.

Physicians and nurses often find it perplexing that Zaner's stories concerning medical ethics are so closely involved with therapy. A family practice physician, after listening to us read a paper on Zaner's therapeutic ethics, had difficulty determining how ethical therapy was distinct from regular medical therapy. He contended that any good physician would do what Zaner did in the story of Tom. He apparently expected us to disagree with him. When we agreed with him, he wanted to know what made ethics distinct from medical care and why an ethicist would be needed in medicine. He seemed to think that an ethicist is a specialist who could be called in to take over moral problems, as an oncologist would be called in when cancer was suspected. Zaner finds being called an ethicist in this context amusing. When his philosophical colleagues ask him what he has become, he says with a wry smile, "I am an ethicist." Zaner's amusement stems from his belief that he is not a specialist in the sense that an oncologist is. Moral decisions are the most common and essential decisions human beings make. The family physician was right in contending that a good physician should help patients understand how treatments relate to their beliefs, values, and aspirations for the good life. From our conversation with him, we had no doubt that this was what he considered good medical practice. The fact that he had traveled from South Africa to The Netherlands to participate in a conference on the human sciences indicated that he was an unusual physician. He believed, as we do, that moral considerations are an essential part of therapy. Therefore, he took it for granted that physicians would be concerned with helping patients make morally right decisions. Ethicists should not take over therapeutic ethics from health care professionals. Instead, they should help them to recognize the ethical considerations inherent in therapy and to engage in therapeutic ethics more adequately.

An example of cooperative therapeutic ethics engaged in by an ethicist and a nurse is given in one of the stories in Zaner's book (1993). In the story entitled "If You Don't Ask, You Won't Know," a nurse works with Zaner to formulate a plan of future treatment for a patient who seems to have no family or advanced directive. The nurse initiated this cooperation and was the primary source of information that came from interaction with the patient.

Mrs. French was a patient in the post-surgical intensive care unit after an exploratory laparotomy had shown that she had a massive abdominal infection and an eight-centimeter aortic aneurysm. Her nurse, Susan Ramat, asked Zaner to talk with Dr. Tray, Mrs. French's attending physician, about her situation. When Zaner asked why he should talk with Dr. Tray, Susan explained the situation.

"'I'm not altogether sure. I just have a feeling that . . . well, so far as we know, she doesn't have any family, and she's really in a bad way now. Things could get worse, too, in a hurry.'

'Really? Why is that?'

'She was brought into a hospital in her hometown with a swollen belly and very high fever, then transferred here for exploratory abdominal surgery. When she was opened up, they found widespread infection. They were able to clean her up a lot, but then discovered an eight-centimeter aneurysm, a triple A, which couldn't be corrected because of all the infection.'

An eight-centimeter abdominal aortic aneurysm—good lord, I thought, that's about as big as my fist! 'If it breaks or leaks, she's really going to be in bad trouble,' I remarked. 'And she has no family, at all?'

'Not so far as we know,' Susan replied. 'The thing is, Dr. Zaner, that she could get into trouble really quickly, and there's just nobody who can speak for her, make decisions, tell us about her wishes, nobody.'

'She has no advance directive?'

'Not that we've found,' Susan said. 'Look in the chart, right there, on the intake form. See? It's left blank where "Living Will" is listed.'

'Do you think you or her nurse could ask her about that right now? She seems alert; maybe she could tell us about that. I mean, if she does have a living will, we'd better know about it, right? Even more, if she's signed a Durable Power of Attorney for Health Decisions, we'll have to get ahold of her attorney-in-fact.'" (Zaner 1993, 120–121)

Zaner discovered that she was admitted by a friend, Mr. Broadmor, and her brother, from whom she was estranged, had given permission for the surgery. Eventually, by asking questions, Zaner and Susan discovered that Mrs. French also had a father and mother, a sister, and five children—all of whom were so estranged from her that they would be of little help in giving moral and legal directives if her situation worsened.

Given her family situation, Zaner thought that he should question Mrs. French about her living will.

"'Mrs. French, you indicated to Susan yesterday that you have a living will, but your friend Mr. Broadmor, can't find it at your home, where you said it was . . .' Before I could continue, her eyes recoiled in utter fear. She whipped her head over to Susan on the other side of the bed, pleading, her hands flailing out, tears beginning to brim out.

And Susan, bless her, immediately began soothing, calming, reassuring her that, no, she wasn't dying. Soon, Susan was able to ask her about the living will. Mrs. French again nodded that she did have one. When Susan asked where she kept it, as it wasn't where her friend could find it, Mrs. French managed eventually to indicate that maybe it was with her attorney back in her hometown.

While Susan continued to comfort and reassure her, I slunk out of the room, deeply embarrassed at my blunder. Obviously, I needed to creep up on the question, needed to realize that in her condition *of course* the first thing she'd think about when quizzed about the living will would be *her* death. I just scared her. That it was unintentional was hardly enough. That I had thought that, having already discussed it yesterday, she would of course be able to discuss it today was also a paltry excuse for the blunder, or at least so I saw it.

I managed to relate what had happened to Mr. Broadmor. He knew her attorney and gave me the phone number. I explained and apologized for my blunder. He was kind, then said he'd like to go in to see her. When Susan came out, wondering why I had left the room, I explained to her.

'Nonsense,' she said, 'she's just having a hard time, and her pain is really awful. I don't think you goofed.'

'Well, I do,' I replied. 'Anyway, I'll get back in to see her later on and apologize for frightening her. Right now, I need to call that attorney and find out about this living will business— finally, I hope!'" (Zaner 1993, 128–129)

From her lawyer, Zaner discovered that she merely had a regular will, making Mr. Broadmor the executor of her estate. This enabled Zaner to make the necessary arrangements to carry out Mrs. French's wishes concerning future operations, treatments, and terminal care when and if they became necessary. Zaner mused, "From thinking that she had 'no family' but that she did have a 'living will,' we learned over the span of a mere three days that she *did* indeed have a family and *no* living will. None of this would have been known if she hadn't been asked" (135).

From *Troubled Voices: Stories of Ethics and Illness* by Richard Zaner. Copyright 1993 by Richard M. Zaner, Jr. Cleveland, Ohio: Pilgrim Press. Used with permission.

Susan initiated the asking that led Zaner to query the attending physician, the attorney, and Mr. Broadmor. In addition, Susan was the only person who asked Mrs. French directly about her family, situation, and living will, except for Zaner's blundered attempt. Her concern for the well-being of her patient and of the staff seems to have been more moral than legal, although it was probably both. She wanted her patient to be able to give direction for her care if the situation worsened. She also seemed concerned that her patient could be left to face these decisions alone without friend or family. With Zaner's help, she discovered that Mrs. French was left alone by a large family but had a close personal friend. This friend was encouraged to see her and take part in her plans. Susan and Zaner were concerned with fostering Mrs. French's well-being within the context of her situation. Most of their activity, however, was directed at her future care, especially concerning her wishes for care if her situation worsened. She became better and was released until she was able to undergo an operation for the aneurysm.

Most health care ethics is directed at a future that cannot be assured in advance. For example, Susan and Zaner were making provisions for what could happen. All therapy is future-oriented and is contingent. This is why, earlier in the book, we said that physicians and nurses, and now ethicists, act "as if," that is, they act as if what they are doing will benefit the patient. These actions are intended to be therapeutic. The ethical actions of Susan and Zaner were therapeutic, in that they were taken as if they would foster Mrs. French's well-being by helping future caregivers to know her wishes and to be able to act therapeutically with dispatch.

If Susan had had time to do so, she could have helped Mrs. French formulate a directive for her future care, as Zaner did. Also, most nurses could have helped Tom discover what would have made an even more dependent life worth living. In fact, nurses are usually better situated and prepared by experience, education, and disposition than most physicians to be involved in therapeutic ethics. Nursing therapy involves ethical considerations that most nurses are capable of dealing with. They may need help from an ethicist to prepare them to recognize the moral aspects of nursing care and to assist them with especially difficult cases. Most cases in nursing ethics books focus on exceptionally difficult cases, but most moral decisions made by nurses concern issues that do not require the assistance of ethicists to resolve. Nurses need to be taught to recognize and articulate these issues as moral ones. One major function of ethicists is to disclose the moral in health care situations, as Zaner does in his recent book.

Since Zaner primarily discloses the ethical in medical therapy, we will attempt such disclosure in cases involving nursing care. Often the ethical in therapeutic situations is disclosed in relationships of caring presence with patients in extremely difficult situations. These cases concern how to care in difficult situations, rather than how to solve difficult moral problems. In the story of Lara, as told by her nurse, Robin Kramer, nurses reached out with compassion to Lara and her family and helped them live fully in the face of Lara's impending death.

"Lara, as I intuitively expected, was a bright-eyed, blond four-teen-year-old girl who, despite her illness, managed to smile and show a spunky personality at our first meeting. She was trying to be brave, but the fear in her eyes was undeniable. I introduced myself as the pediatric oncology clinical nurse specialist and began to orient Lara and her family to the Medical Center of the University of California at San Francisco. I explained that my role was to inform them about diagnostic tests that would occur over the next few days, to educate them about the disease and treatment once the diagnosis was confirmed, to coordinate Lara's medical and nursing care, to act as a liaison to the medical staff, fielding concerns and grievances, to help in any way possible, and to just be a friend during this frightening experience.

"I assured Lara and her family that although UCSF is a large medical center, Lara's care would be individualized. She would not be just 'another patient' or 'a case study' to us, but a very important person. She and her family would be the focus of our care. I also reassured the family that because UCSF is a large medical center, we have access to the latest knowledge and technology.

"Over the next two days, while waiting for confirmation of the diagnosis, I did a lot of listening. I heard about the symptoms and events that had led to Lara's hospitalization. I listened to the expression of shock, fear, and guilt—how could this diagnosis of leukemia be possible? The nursing staff and I spent considerable time getting to know Lara and her family—their coping strengths, their weaknesses, who supports whom and how. We did not negate their concerns or try to offer false assurance. We acknowledged their feelings as real and helped the family sort through them in a healthy and meaningful way.

"It was clear to all involved that one of the most useful things we could do for this distraught family, who was in a strange and overwhelming place, was to assist them, little by little, in gaining control over their experiences. This involved helping them anticipate and be prepared for what was to come, for how it might feel or look physically and emotionally. It also involved helping them to continue in their usual roles as much as possible and engaging them as appropriate in the decisions affecting Lara's care. The sincerity conveyed to the family convinced them that someone would always be there for them during the low times." (Benner and Wrubel 1989, 298–299)

Kramer and the nursing staff structured Lara's care to meet her concerns during her eight weeks of hospitalization. They secured a telephone for her so that she could call her friends. Kramer followed Lara's lead in her care of Lara—sometimes they joked, sometimes listened to music, and at other times they talked about serious issues. Kramer nonverbally indicated to Lara that it was all right to be angry or depressed. Kramer and the staff arranged a birthday party for Lara, and Kramer took Lara and two friends on a Sunday outing in her car.

In spite of medical treatment and nursing care, Lara's prognosis continued to grow dimmer. When Lara and her family considered a bone marrow transplant (BMT), her nurses arranged for a young woman who had had a BMT to come to talk to Lara. In discussing the possibilities of a BMT with Lara and her family, Kramer did not temper their enthusiasm with the negative side of BMT. When there was no match for BMT within the family, Kramer took the opportunity to explain the unpleasant side of BMT and acknowledge the gamut of emotions evoked when certain decisions are out of one's control.

The ability to control Lara's condition lessened. Lara started to have high fevers, seemed tired despite transfusions, and needed oxygen. At Kramer's suggestion, Lara's mother called the family together to be with Lara in her final hours.

"Lara needed to be intubated because her respiratory status continued to deteriorate. This was a terrible experience for her; she continuously gestured to us to remove the tube. The medical and nursing staff, along with Lara's family, acknowledged that Lara's death was imminent. Our greatest gift to Lara would be to give back her dignity by removing the respirator. She immediately started talking in a high, squeaky voice, and plans quickly developed to have a party 'to toast Lara's awakening,' as Joann aptly described it.

"As I visited with Lara, she looked me directly in the eyes and said, 'I'm so sick, am I going to die?' Although it was a matter of seconds before I answered, it seemed like hours as my mind groped for the right words. I did not avert my gaze and answered from my heart: 'I'm frightened Lara, you are so sick that you could die. I know you must be terribly scared, too. Everyone you love is with you, and we won't leave.' She nodded and quietly closed her eyes to rest. Shortly thereafter, the champagne arrived, and we toasted Lara—her extubation, her courage, and her spirit. She smiled and said, 'I love you all very much.'" Two hours later, she died peacefully with her family nearby. (Benner and Wrubel 1989, 301–302)

Kramer not only cared for Lara but for her family as well. Lara's mother commented, "Any degree of stability I was able to maintain over the next eight weeks was due largely to the unwavering support and encouragement of this dedicated young woman. Her daily concern was not only for the patient but for each family member" (Benner and Wrubel 1989, 304).

The foregoing is both an example of excellent nursing and of therapeutic ethics. A therapeutic ethics is one in which the values of the patient and the response of the nurse to those values are integrally involved in patient therapy. The response of Kramer, and indeed the whole health care staff, to Lara's situation was one of affiliation and compassion. Lara's situation brought a response from her nurses that made evident the moral sense that often goes unnoticed in all health care. The only "big" ethical decision in Lara's care concerned removing the respirator. Yet in the story, it did not appear as a big decision but merely as the continuation of a pervasive ongoing way of caring for Lara that helped her to live her last days as well as possible. Everyday moral decisions concerned making arrangements for her to phone her friends, arranging a birthday party for her, and making special arrangements for a trip on the town with some of her friends. Some of the contributions of nurses to Lara's living as well as possible were mentioned after her death by her mother: one nurse braided Lara's hair to delay and, in her case, prevent baldness; another nurse attempted to take her to a concert and when that was not possible brought her a full report and memorabilia from the concert; another shared her tapes with Lara and talked with her about the music Lara liked (Benner and Wrubel 1989, 303–306).

When caring for fourteen year olds, discovering the way that they want to live the remainder of their lives rarely comes from philosophical discussions of the meaning of life. In Lara's case, it came from her nurses, and especially Kramer, from being with her and discovering what gave meaning to her life—conversing with friends, listening to music, escaping from the hospital, having parties, being attractive, and, above all, being surrounded by caring people who loved her and whom she loved. Lara's nurses disclosed to Lara and her family that their care *of* her really expressed their care *for* her.

Another example of such care is evident in the home care given by Barbara to a man whose situation was quite different from Lara's. He seemed to have little to live for, having lost his wife, his twin brother, his business, and his independence. Now facing the loss of his health, from congestive heart failure, and his dependence on continuous nursing care, he felt that his life had little meaning.

One day, upon one of my home visits as I was assessing him and engaging him in conversation, he began to cry again. Having built a rapport with him, and feeling I had gained his trust, I put down my stethoscope, got down on my knees by the side of his chair and took his hand in mine.... I knelt there holding his hand and quietly listening, and then I shared with him how much he had come to mean to me—that knowing him had enriched my life—that he was a very special person. A bond was forged that day. A bond of trust, understanding, and caring. It is a bond that continues to grow as I continue to care for this patient with all of those losses and chronic needs that impact his daily life.

What struck me the most was that it was not my stethoscope or my teaching that impacted him the most, but simply *time*— time to talk, to touch, and to care.

In the foregoing case, the relationship of therapy and morality is so intertwined that it would be difficult to separate one from the other. The nurse discovered that her patient's well-being required much more than ordinary assessment and care. In dialogue she realized that her patient's emptiness came from a loss of almost everything that gave his life meaning and a sense of worth. Her personal way of being with him helped restore meaning and worth to his life.

Barbara's personal relationship with her patient was enhanced by meeting him on his level. This was literally true in the case of her kneeling down to be beside him in his chair. Kay Toombs (1992), a philosopher with multiple sclerosis, tells how posture and speech affect ill and debilitated persons. She is irritated by people who ignore her by directing questions to her husband and referring to her in the third person when she is in a wheelchair. "Would *she* like to sit at this table?" "What would *she* like to drink?" (65). She recounts being wheeled up to a security barrier in an airport, where the attendant turned to her husband and said, "Can *she* walk at all?" Her husband retorted, "Yes, and she can talk, too!" (136). Toombs contends that autonomy is directly related to the ability to assume an upright posture. She says, "To be able to 'stand on one's own two feet' is of more than figurative significance" (65). Toombs discloses how demeaning some spatial terms used to refer to the ill can be.

> There is more than metaphorical significance to such expressions as "to look down on," and "to look up to." In the hospital setting the patient, more often than not, is in bed and must "look up to" the doctor who "stands" talking and "looking down on" the patient. In "looking up to" the doctor, and "being looked down on," the patient feels on an unequal "footing" with the physician, concretely diminished in autonomy. . . . In this regard it is worth noting that patients are likely to feel much less "inferior" if the physician sits down by the bedside, so that they are on the same level ("eye to eye") when communicating with one another. (Toombs 1992, 65–66)

The way in which nurses posture themselves in relationship to patients and speak of their lived spatial relationships with them is of import in therapeutic ethics. Posture and speech can deny or assure patients their autonomy, and make evident the extent of their nurses' concern for them and involvement with them.

In the foregoing cases, both Barbara and Kramer establish a relationship with their patients that fosters their well-being and enhances their zest for life. In both cases, being compassionately called to care by the plight of another person appears to be more important than exceptional nursing skill or knowledge. Using such cases to illustrate the meaning of therapeutic ethics has the danger of reinforcing an unfortunate misunderstanding of the meaning of the moral in nursing. It can imply that morality in nursing concerns going the extra mile outside of and detached from nursing care. In both of the above cases the nurses go the extra mile, but in a direction called for by excellent nursing practice. Put differently, both nurses fulfill the moral sense of nursing by moving beyond competent care to excellent care in order to foster their patients' well-being.

An example of therapeutic ethics that is less concerned with going the extra mile in personal relations, and that involves the integral relationship of moral, personal, technical, and practical care, is the case of Mr. Jones. In this case his nurse, Mary Cucci, skillfully restored Mr. Jones to his lived body after he had lost the ability to live in and through his body, out of fear resulting from the repeated firings of an implanted defibrillator and from cardiac arrests.

"The night of his admission, . . . he had been 'automatically' defibrillated twenty times in the period of an hour before an intravenous medication could control the rhythm.

I first met Mr. Jones the morning after his admission to the CCU. The nurse on the previous shift told me about the terror he had been through. He had screamed with the repeated defibrillation, had required a significant amount of sedation, and had been rambling and panicky until the sedation took effect.

As I entered the room, . . . his eyes focused on me, but the rest of his body seemed frozen in the bed. His body was limp and his muscles looked wasted as if he had lost considerable weight. We had a brief, quiet conversation of introduction. . . . I told him that I understood that he had been through a great deal. I asked him gently if he would tell me how he felt about it. He replied:

'How would you feel? It was a nightmare.' As he continued to speak, his face began to reflect his pain and anxiety. His eyes began to tear. His voice was tremulous and frail. . . . 'What am I going to do now? I thought this (the implanted defibrillator) was the last answer. What if it happened again? I couldn't stand that'. . . .

I told him that I would help him find some answers, and that I was going to help him through this. I shared my impressions of him; that he appeared overwhelmed, with a million thoughts running through his mind at once, and that he seemed to feel as if he felt out of control. He said, 'Yes, that is how I feel.' He seemed surprised that somehow I understood. He also talked about feeling betrayed by the device that was supposed to be the answer. He talked about his fear of it happening again. I discussed Mr. Jones's distress with his physicians and encouraged them to discuss the possibility of turning off the defibrillator while he was in the CCU. By two in the afternoon, with Mr. Jones's approval, the defibrillator was turned off. . . .

Despite the emotional and intellectual intensity he displayed, Mr. Jones moved minimally in the bed. This intense man appeared trapped in a frozen shell. Some of it was due to the debilitation of his weight loss and recent illnesses, but as I began talking to him about moving more and maintaining and building his physical strength, I began to realize he was afraid to move. He admitted it. Apparently, several of his tachycardias had occurred during exertion. This time I persisted and after an explanation of the importance of moving his arms, legs, and body gently around in the bed, he began to make some progress. Suddenly he was aware of every premature heartbeat he had. I told him when he was right and when he was wrong. We watched the monitor together. We set up a plan for increased mobility and negotiated each limit. I stayed with him through each new step. It was like watching someone wake up physically, but the process was slower and more obviously sequential. It was the mental hurdle we were really facing. I challenged him to meet the goals we set. I distracted him with conversation. He watched the clock ferociously and met his goal with not a minute extra given. He began moving more in the bed without thinking about it. More of his body participated as he continued to talk of the intense emotional issues he faced. I teased him, cajoled him, and danced with him as he transferred to the chair. I challenged him more each day and ignored his fake whine when he half-heartedly pleaded abuse. It became a joke. He learned to monitor his pulse to guide his activity progression. This was a long, slow process of building belief in himself. I told him throughout that I knew it was difficult, that I admired his strength, and that I knew he could do it." (Benner and Wrubel 1989, 247–250)

Through dialogue with Mr. Jones, Cucci discovered that he had never really confronted the likelihood of his own death and that he had lived a life that was so ordered that he even followed a diagram for each day's work. Now he could not plan or order his life and was confronted with the fear of death. He commented, "This time everything has been taken away," to which Cucci responded that his wife, who had faithfully supported him, had not been taken away. He responded, "If it wasn't for her, I don't know what I would do." (Benner and Wrubel 1989, 248).

"Several months after discharge, Mr. Jones and his wife returned to the CCU to say hello. We greeted each other with hugs and smiles. He had gained weight and I teased him about his potbelly. Eight months after discharge he is still doing well and reports to his physician that he is feeling better and better." (Benner and Wrubel 1989, 250).

From *The Primacy of Caring: Stress and Coping in Health and Disease* by Patricia Benner and Judith Wrubel. Copyright 1989. Menlo Park, Cal.: Addison-Wesley. Used with permission of Mary Cucci.

The goal of therapy is to foster the well-being of the patient, and, thus, it is to fulfill the moral sense of health care. Ethics is concerned with how well the moral sense is fulfilled. In the above story, Cucci helps foster the well-being of Mr. Jones by engrossment in his situation and by dialogue that assures him that his response to his illness and treatment is understandable and acceptable, and that she is willing to act on his behalf. She shares Mr. Jones's fears with his physician, and they agree, with Mr. Jones's permission, to terminate the defibrillator. Termination of the machine leads him to face his own mortality and to raise the question of whether or not he is committing suicide. Since Cucci feels inadequate to deal with this question, she refers him to a chaplain for consultation. She also seeks the assistance of a psychiatric nurse to help him deal with the disruptions in his life that he is so ill-prepared to handle. She personally helps him to understand that his relationship with his wife is a source of meaning and assurance. Perhaps her greatest contribution is the tactful, resourceful, and compassionate way in which she helps him overcome his fear of bodily movement and her skill, sensitivity, and persistence in helping him learn to relive his body within the constraints of new circumstances.

The fearful response of Mr. Jones to his situation shows us how illness can alienate us from our body and how it can restrict our space. Mr. Jones was literally afraid to move and was virtually imprisoned in a strange body that he feared. He could not move because of fear that movement would trigger tachycardia. Although his fear was exaggerated, it was not unwarranted. He had to learn bodily movement because his physical well-being required movement. Cucci helped him to learn to move in ways that overcame his fear by using a monitor. It is important, however, to recognize that he was not learning to move according to the monitor but according to his lived experience of his body. The monitor merely gave him assurance and set limits that came to be recognized by the lived body. Eventually, he was able to move within these limits even when Cucci deliberately distracted him from being overtly conscious of his body.

Cucci contributed to his physical well-being by fostering the movement that his body required to heal. To do this she worked with his lived body. He had to learn to relive his body, not just for his physical well-being, but for his personal well-being. Toombs (1992) observes that "to address the patient's experiences of disorder, attention must be paid not only to the physical manifestation of a disease state but also to the changing relations between body, self, and world" (82). She contends that chronic illness in particular requires giving attention to "essential features" of "embodiment . . . such as being-in-the-world, bodily intentionality, . . . body image, gestural display" and lived space and time (82). These aspects of embodiment are evident in Mr. Jones's case. How can he be in a world in which everything is not controlled and he is not autonomous? His former bodily intentionality presupposed an ordered world in which his lived body functioned autonomously and reliably. His image of his body had to undergo a major transformation from that of control, order, and autonomy to that of a body subject to natural forces over which he had little control. His gestural display, rather than being a display of power and self-assurance, became one of fear, uncertainty, and withdrawal. His space, which once was open and invited autonomous movement, had become not only confined to a bed but to a strange body. He seemed to have no future because he could not project himself beyond the body into which he had retreated. Then Cucci taught him how to live that body again. Instead of being a frightened stranger confined to a body that he occupied and feared, he once again became confidently embodied in the world.

When he returned several months later and greeted and hugged Cucci, Mr. Jones's gestural display was that of a fully embodied person reaching out to embrace those for whom he cared. Cucci reported that eight months later he felt better and that his "amiodarone had been reduced and no significant arrhythmias recurred" (Benner 1987, 172). Strangely, she omitted that he seemed to have become an embodied person living well with self, others, and world.

One aspect of therapy deals with treatment that cures or improves bodily function: "amiodarone had been reduced and no significant arrhythmias recurred." This refers primarily to the body as a biological machine. Ethics is important to this aspect of health care to ensure that technology is encased in its original moral intent—for the good of the other. The other aspect concerns the lived body interacting with self, others, and world. Concern for the well-being of the lived body is the focus of therapeutic ethics. For example, Tom's physicians focused on the body object—dialysis will keep it alive. Zaner focused on the lived body and world by asking why Tom should want to live or die.

Cucci did not overtly address the philosophical question Mr. Jones asked, concerning whether a life that could not be strictly ordered and controlled was worth living. Instead, she answered this question practically with her care for Mr. Jones. She obviously believed, as did Mr. Jones after he recovered from his fears, that it is good to be embodied and live your body in relationship to self, others, and the world. Cucci concretely engaged in therapeutic relationships and actions that restored Mr. Jones to his lived body in relationship to self, others, and world. She moved him from entombment in his body to timid movement while meter watching, and finally to dancing, in restoring him to the world that he so obviously enjoyed *being* in during their last meeting. Cucci's nursing therapy that fosters the well-being of Mr. Jones's lived body in relationship to self, others, and world is an example of therapeutic ethics in practice. There are two kinds of therapy. One is a mechanistic therapy that treats the anatomical body as a machine to be fixed and controlled with machines, chemicals, and surgery. The purpose of the implanted defibrillator was to regulate the functioning of Mr. Jones's heart. The machine's failure not only concerned the anatomical body but Mr. Jones's lived body. The machine was not experienced by Mr. Jones as a failed heart regulator but as pain that must cease. Cucci engaged in therapeutic ethics when she placed the mechanistic therapy within the context of the lived body by having the machine disconnected. The second therapy directly concerns how the body is lived in relationship to self, others, and world. Cucci engaged in therapeutic ethics directly when her care in practical ways helped Mr. Jones face and answer questions related to his illness and debilitation. Mr. Jones's anxiety about future pain focused his attention on his lived body's relationship to the self. How can he become confident and assertive when he is under the constant threat of pain? His apprehension about lack of order and autonomy focused his concern on his lived body's relationship to the world. How can he live the ordered life required in business when his lived body makes his world unpredictable and unreliable? His recognition of the importance of his wife focused his concern on the importance of his lived body to others. How can he refuse to undergo the therapy needed to restore his health when his wife is so important to him and dependent upon him? A therapeutic ethics is focused on the lived world and how wellness, illness, debilitation, and treatment affect the lived body's relation to self, others, and the world. Ethics is therapeutic when it helps nurses foster the well-being of the whole person as he/she projects himself/herself in the world. By so doing, it keeps nursing focused on its primary and inherent moral purpose—fostering the well-being of the other—and on the therapeutic caring presence through which that purpose is fulfilled.

Study Questions

1. What does Zaner mean by clinical ethics? Why do Anne and Jack believe that his ethics should be called a therapeutic ethics?
2. Drawing on the story of Tom, give an interpretation of therapeutic ethics. If you had been Tom's nurse, how would you have engaged in therapeutic ethics? Give an example of your own engagement in therapeutic ethics, from your experience of nursing. If your experience is limited, give an imaginary example.
3. What moral issue is involved in the case of Susan and Zaner's care for Mrs. French? If you had encountered this case in a text that was not called an ethics book, would you have recognized the moral issues involved? If not, what does your failure to recognize the moral issues in this case of everyday care indicate about the way some nurses think about ethics?
4. Why is the nursing care of Lara by Kramer and other nurses an example of therapeutic ethics? Describe other examples of nursing care in which the morality of nurses involved quality care in difficult situations, rather than difficult moral issues to be resolved.

5. What do the case of Barbara and the experience of Kay Toombs indicate about how the posture of nurses in relating to patients is involved in therapeutic ethics?
6. Discuss the ethical questions Mr. Jones and Cucci faced in his nursing care. Why do Anne and Jack contend that Cucci answered some of the questions practically rather than theoretically?
7. How does Kay Toombs's analysis of how illness changes relationships between lived body and self, others, and world enlighten what Mr. Jones is experiencing?
8. Describe how Cucci helps Mr. Jones learn to relive his body. Give an example of how you have helped or might help patients learn to relive their bodies or some function of their bodies, such as grasping or walking.
9. Why does Cucci's report that Mr. Jones felt "better and better" and that his "amiodarone had been reduced and no significant arrhythmias recurred" fail to do justice to her excellent care? Do you believe that nurses often fail to articulate the full ethical significance of their care? Why or why not?
10. What two kinds of therapy are treated by Jack and Anne? What is the ethical import of each? How are they related to each other? In which is therapeutic ethics most involved? Why?

References

Benner, Patricia, and Judith Wrubel. (1989). *The Primacy of Caring: Stress and Coping in Health and Disease.* Menlo Park, Cal.: Addison-Wesley.

Bishop, Anne H., and John R. Scudder, Jr. (1990). *The Practical, Moral, and Personal Sense of Nursing: A Phenomenological Philosophy of Practice.* Albany, N.Y. : State University of New York Press.

Toombs, S. Kay. (1992). *The Meaning of Illness: A Phenomenological Account of the Different Perspectives of Physician and Patient.* Dordrecht: Kluwer Academic Publishers.

Veatch, Robert M., and Sara T. Fry. (1987). *Case Studies in Nursing Ethics.* Philadelphia: J. B. Lippincott.

Zaner, Richard M. (1988). *Ethics and the Clinical Encounter.* Englewood Cliffs, N.J.: Prentice Hall.

Zaner, Richard M. (1993). *Troubled Voices: Stories of Ethics and Illness.* Cleveland, Ohio: Pilgrim Press.

6

Reflexive Dialogue on
Ethics and Nursing

Ethics is integrally related to nursing, because nursing is a practice with an inherent moral sense. Nursing ethics attempts to articulate that moral sense, to assess its fulfillment, to explore new possibilities for its fulfillment, and to appraise its adequacy. These articulations, appraisals, and explorations focus on nursing as practiced, especially on exemplars of nursing excellence. Exemplars both disclose the meaning of *good* nursing care and call nurses into relationships of therapeutic caring presence with patients.

In this work we have interpreted nursing ethics in the four ways implied by the titles of the preceding four chapters. Chapter 2 investigated the meaning of being a good nurse by showing that care as practice and care as concern are integrally related to each other in good care. When nurses are attentive, efficient, and effective in their practice, they are being morally good persons, because they are fulfilling the moral sense of nursing by fostering the well-being of patients. Being concerned about their patients' well-being is built into the practice and presupposed by it. Ethics not only contributes understanding of these two senses of good and how they relate to each other, but it also engages in critical appraisal of how well nursing fulfills its moral sense. This will become more evident in our dialogical interpretation of Margie as an exemplar of being a good nurse.

In Chapter 3, we attempted to describe caring presence drawing on Buber, Noddings, and Zaner. The relationship of ethics to caring presence is so evident that the ethical in nursing is often identified with caring presence. The reason for the tendency to identify the ethical in nursing with caring presence is apparent in the relationship of Beverly and Midori. Caring presence affirms the humanity of both nurse and patient and accords each the respect due a human being. It comforts and supports those cared-for as they face suffering, treatment, and possible death, and at the same time it inspires and enlightens the caregiver.

112

In Chapter 4, we treated nursing as a calling by exploring the meaning of being called to care and philosophical interpretations that enlighten and heighten that call. We rejected the separation typical of Western thought in which call is thought of as motive divorced from meaning and practice. Then, with help from Chinn and Lashley, we showed that the call to care and the meaning of that care are integrally related to each other. Nursing ethics is concerned with understanding and evoking the call to care. In addition, it attempts to situate this calling in a context of the meaning of being human, as we attempted to do by combining Marx's ethics of compassion and Taylor's interpretation of an ethics of authenticity.

In Chapter 5, we showed that nursing ethics, although more adequately interpreted as a clinical ethics than as an applied philosophical ethics, is better understood as a therapeutic ethics. The intent of both therapy and nursing practice is to foster the well-being of the client. Ethics attempts to critique and foster fulfillment of the intent of nursing therapy. But the role of ethics in therapy is not the same for all therapy. Ethics is involved with that aspect of therapy that is primarily technical and biological only to ensure that the technical fulfills its purpose of fostering the well-being of persons and that their rights are respected. Ethics is integrally involved in therapy that concerns the lived body's relationship to self, others, world, and the life projects of persons. That ethics explores the relationship of illness and treatment to the lived body and personal projects is evident in Zaner's work as an ethicist and in our interpretation of the case of Cucci and Mr. Jones.

Although our approach to nursing ethics should be of interest to ethicists, our book is primarily intended for nurses and nursing students. Our purpose has not been to show how ethics can be applied to nursing. Instead, we have shown how the moral sense of nursing impacts on nursing ethics. We want to make nurses aware of the moral import of their practice and how they can better fulfill its moral sense. We hope to encourage them to explore new possibilities by developing new ways to empower their care and by developing visions of the good that will direct their caring practice.

Helping nurses to recognize, fulfill, and enhance the moral sense of nursing requires getting down to cases. Consequently, we will conclude by exploring the meaning and implications for nursing ethics of the exemplars of being a good nurse, of caring presence, and of therapeutic ethics that we have previously discussed. In keeping with the exploratory nature of this interpretation, we will engage in a reflexive dialogue to disclose the meaning of each case for nursing ethics. Most of our writing comes from reflexive dialogue in which we attempt to ferret out the meaning of nursing, to place that meaning within a wider human context, and to explore new possibilities for enhancing nursing practice. We invite the reader to share in our reflexive dialogue.

Reflexive Dialogue

Anne: I always feel more adequate when I attempt to point out how the good is fostered in concrete nursing cases than when I attempt to justify calling what I do nursing ethics.

Jack: You know how I feel about "Is this really X?" questions in philosophy. I remember when a young scholar challenged a leading phenomenologist by asking him if the paper he had read was *really* phenomenology. The philosopher responded, "I've never really thought about it, but I do work out of that tradition and I think I gave an adequate treatment of the philosophical issue with which I was concerned." Like him, I'm much more concerned with articulating and fostering the good inherent in nursing practice than in answering the question, "Is what we're doing *really* ethics?"

Anne: Yes, but this is a book on nursing ethics and we must be as clear as we can about what the stories we have included have to do with ethics.

Jack: If our examples have been well-chosen, their ethical import should be evident. Paul Ricoeur's brief definition of phenomenology is that it is a philosophy primarily concerned with disclosing meaning, that meaning is given as essence, and that essence is disclosed through well-chosen examples (Ricoeur, 1977). Interpretation helps clarify the meaning disclosed through examples and places them in a wider context of meaning.

Being a Good Nurse

Anne: We entitled Chapter 2 "On Being a Good Nurse" because we wanted to explore the meaning of being a good nurse without talking about The Nurse. Margie Smith's story of her care for Mrs. Cooper is an example of outstanding nursing. She becomes so engrossed in Mrs. Cooper's life situation that she recognizes that Mrs. Cooper's determination and courage outweigh the dismal prospects for prostheses for most persons of her age and health status. In her practice, Margie goes to great lengths to foster the well-being of Mrs. Cooper. She engages in a prolonged confrontation with the physician and the physical therapist. She elicits the help of occupational therapists, the clinical nurse specialist, and other staff nurses to prevent Mrs. Cooper's early discharge, to secure two new prostheses, and to arrange for the help necessary for her to learn to walk with them. This is an example of good nursing, but won't some ethicists question its inclusion in an ethics book?

Jack: The story of Margie and Mrs. Cooper should help nurses recognize excellent practice and evoke good nursing care from them. Since nursing practice is designed to foster patient well-being, the reason for its inclusion seems obvious to me. But I realize that in this age of technical philosophy, some ethicists are apt to want more philosophical justification for inclusion of our exemplars in an ethics book. To question inclusion of a story in an ethics book that encourages moral excellence seems odd! Margie is Mrs. Cooper's existential advocate in the sense of Gadow's (1980) interpretation. She helps Mrs. Cooper discover and fulfill the meaning of her life in light of her illness, debilitation, and treatment.

Anne: By now, most nurses have some grasp of the meaning of Gadow's existential advocacy, but doesn't Margie extend the meaning of advocacy beyond Gadow?

Jack: I think I can disclose the further meaning of her advocacy with an example. A friend of mine came to a lecture late and, not wanting to interrupt the proceedings, sat on the floor in the back of the meeting hall. Someone tapped him on the shoulder and said, "Would you be my advocate?" He turned and saw a man on crutches who immediately responded to his puzzled look by asking, "Would you help me find a seat?" Later the two discussed the meaning of advocacy, and the man with the crutches explained that an advocate is someone who helps you do what you cannot do without help, but does so in a way that liberates you from limitations imposed by your disability.

Anne: Margie fulfills that sense of advocacy. The moral sense of nursing pervades her advocacy of Mrs. Cooper. But I'm not sure that she explicitly recognizes the moral imperative inherent in nursing practice or that she realizes that nursing itself is constituted by that imperative. I am surprised that she sums up her outstanding care for Mrs. Cooper by saying, "I'm pleased that I was able to play an instrumental role in improving the quality of life for this patient," and that she regrets that she couldn't give a better example of "positive team-building." (see page 35)

Jack: How can she say "an instrumental role" and "positive team-building"? "Instrumental role" implies technical proficiency rather than moral excellence. Her language blunts the moral impact of her forceful advocacy. Regardless of the adequacy of her language for conveying the moral sense of nursing, her care discloses it superbly. She is so intent on fostering Mrs. Cooper's well-being that she is willing to take on those who safely follow standard treatments for this type of patient rather than seeking treatment suited to Mrs. Cooper. Margie does this by building a team of defenders of the right who become advocates of Mrs. Cooper.

Anne: That sounds macho to me! If I remember it right, Margie maneuvered through a web of connection and skillfully and sensitively encouraged others to see the right action. She persistently led others to the right action rather than, as you say, demanded that it be done!

Jack: You're right. Her way of caring is well described by Gilligan's feminist ethics. But do not miss the quality of her moral stance by labeling it feminine rather than masculine. She not only forcefully demands that nursing fulfill its moral sense but also calls physicians and other health care workers to live up to a high standard of fostering the well-being of others. That's what is odd about her remark about not giving an example of positive team building. She builds a positive team out of a very unpromising situation.

Anne: It may seem odd to *you* that someone who is so practically and morally on target cannot articulate the meaning of her care, but not to me. Like many nurses, she has been taught to speak in technical language, i.e. "being instrumental," and professional language, i.e. "positive team building," rather than in the moral language common to everyday relationships.

Jack: I may be old-fashioned but I believe that ethics should articulate the moral sense of such admirable actions and interactions. When I was a young scholar, being good and doing good were considered moral, while ethics was the study of and articulation of morality.

Anne: That's the kind of ethics we nurses need to study. I've always felt that nurses were better moral beings than they give themselves credit for. Recently, the lack of recognition of the moral quality of our work has been obscured by the professional and technological language that was so evident in Margie's inadequate articulation of her excellent moral care.

Jack: Nurses not only fail to do justice to the moral quality of their practice, but they often focus on the wrong moral issues. For example, care and rights seem to go together. I'm puzzled by nursing scholars who foster unnecessary conflict between advocates of care and advocates of autonomy and rights.

Anne: You wouldn't be puzzled if you were a woman. Men have always taken advantage of the tendency of women to care and nurture. Although I believe, as you do, that care and rights go together, I can sure understand why many of my colleagues are suspicious that stressing the value of caring might carry with it a denial of rights.

Jack: I think that arguing about care versus rights sidetracks us from the major struggle in health care. The primary battle in health care is between those who believe that the moral sense is the essence of health care practice and those who think that health care practice is essentially application of instrumental reason. Our primary concern should be the place of morality in nursing and not theoretical squabbles predicated on the assumption that morality already has a major place.

Anne: The technocratic and bureaucratic tendencies in nursing obscure the moral sense of nursing. I'm concerned that faith in instrumental reason with its stress on efficiency is leading us away from the moral sense of nursing. What will happen to nursing when stress on efficient instrumental reasoning replaces concern for persons, for their rights, and for being a good person?

Jack: I am more disturbed about *how* personal relationships and rights are incorporated into health care when it is interpreted as instrumental reason. It seems to me that in such an interpretation, concern for personal relationships and for rights can only be tangentially incorporated in therapy. For example, it is often argued that when medical and nursing therapy are interpreted as applied science, we especially need to treat patients as persons and to respect their rights. But this makes concern with personal relationships and rights an adjunct to therapy rather than an integral aspect of therapy.

Anne: But we do need to recognize the place of rights in nursing care.

Jack: Of course, but we need to relate rights appropriately to care. Remember, if Tom's rights had been respected he would have died. What saved his life was Zaner's therapeutic caring presence that helped him find possibilities for a life worth living. I go to the hospital because I need care, not because I want justice or my rights respected. If I need justice, I go to a lawyer, or a judge, or a lawmaker.

Anne: But if nurses did not respect your rights or those of your fellow patients, you would be the first to raise Cain! Nurses need to be just and to respect people's rights. The imbalance of power between nurse and patients makes respecting persons and recognizing their rights imperative.

Jack: But as an integral part of nursing care, not as an adjunct.

Anne: Margie does that beautifully. She shows that being a good nurse and a moral one are integrally related to each other.

Jack: I wish she had been able to articulate the moral worth of what she did more adequately. But that is a contribution to nursing that ethics should make.

Anne: I hope you philosophers recognize that ethics could not make that contribution without examples of moral excellence such as Margie's care for Mrs. Cooper.

Caring Presence: Midori and Beverly

Jack: The relationship of caring presence between Midori and Beverly is an exemplar of moral excellence. Beverly's way of telling the story discloses the moral worth of their relationship.

Anne: I'm amazed that Midori's caring presence for Beverly is what I first recall from the story.

Jack: The caring presence of Midori transforms Beverly's nursing care. Zaner often says that the caring presence of patients is therapeutic for the caregiver. He believes that this aspect of caring is much neglected.

Anne: He puts it more strongly than that. He stresses that caring itself is therapeutic for the caregiver. Remember how Beverly affirmed that caring for Midori made Beverly realize what it *really* means to be a nurse.

Jack:	That's true, but caregiving for some patients is not therapeutic for nurses. In our study of fulfillment in nursing, most of the least fulfilling situations for nurses concerned patients who were uncooperative and unappreciative.
Anne:	That's why caring for patients like Midori has such a therapeutic effect on nurses. When "Midori moments" occur, nursing makes sense and is worthwhile.
Jack:	New possibilities of care are envisioned and a deeper quality of care is evoked.
Anne:	But we have been so captivated by Midori that we have neglected Beverly. I wonder why.
Jack:	Because we expect caring presence from nurses but not patients, especially when they are in pain and facing imminent death.
Anne:	Isn't a good nurse one who sensitively responds to the caring presence of a person like Midori? One reason we so remember Midori in this story is that Beverly's sensitive description of her makes us aware of what a magnificent person Midori is. In addition, Beverly's response to Midori is so subtle and unobtrusive that its quality is easily unrecognized.
Jack:	Talk about engrossment! Listen to this. "Her breathing was shallow and rapid. With each labored breath, her neck muscles strained and her abdomen protruded. We looked at each other, searching for the right thing to say. Only our tears came. Then silence." (see page 63)
Anne:	I want my nursing students to read that. They need to learn when to be silent. They feel they must help and that talking helps, but often silence helps.
Jack:	But silence helps more in a relationship of co-presence. I am struck by how Beverly and Midori are continually present to each other in speech, in silence, in touch.
Anne:	Such deep relationships of co-presence cannot be created. They can only be evoked and anticipated.

Knowing how to help someone through trying times without intruding or imposing is excellent nursing. Unfortunately, such caring presence is underappreciated as nursing excellence in this day of intervention.

Jack: We have omitted a crucial aspect of caring. Our friend Ingegerd Harder (1993) always stresses that caring presence involves more than personal relationships. It also is apparent in skillful, effective, and efficient care.

Anne: I thought of that when I remembered how Beverly's bathing of Midori relaxed her. Ingegerd's example of the bath combined the personal with skillful, effective, and efficient nursing care. It is amazing how often caring presence is evident in bathing. Nurses lose an opportunity for tactile presence when they delegate bathing to assistive personnel.

Jack: I've always thought of bathing as something that anyone could do, but in Ingegerd's example, bathing appeared to me as a high level skill in nursing.

Anne: It can be. Remember how the patient said it seemed to her that the nurse had been doing this for a hundred years? In our technological age, we think of skilled care as involving gadgets and knowledge derived from science. This nurse's knowledge and skill came from nursing experience—her own and that of others who came before her.

Jack: I was impressed by the nurse's I-Thou relationship with the patient. Listen to the patient's description of the bathing. "She had a special way of helping in concrete ways like washing my back and feet, which I could not reach that morning. 'I suggest that you' . . . and 'what you could do is turning your body. . .' yes she was assisting me, never taking over. I was in command, I felt. I mattered. Even though the only thing I could manage was steering the shower handle." (see page 40)

Anne: That's real caring presence. In this relationship it's by empowering the patient, encouraging her, and giving her hope that the nurse tells the patient that she matters.

Jack: Caring presence makes you know that you really
         matter. That's why it's important to understand the
         place of caring presence in affirming a person's
         worth. We philosophers attempt to do that by
         arguments that assign persons to a status or place
         them in a category, but a real felt sense that affirms
         your worth comes from experiencing caring
         presence.

Anne: Until now, I've never thought of intimate hands-on
         care as a way of affirming the worth of a person. But
         I've always thought that intimate relationships are at
         the heart of nursing. Others must feel the same way,
         since the ethical in nursing is so often identified with
         caring presence.

Called to Care

Jack: I am sure that I'm not called to care in the tactile,
         intimate way that you nurses are.

Anne: Your caring usually involves thinking. I've learned
         from you that I can care by thinking. We nurses
         seem to dissociate thinking about meaning from
         caring. We do believe that instrumental reasoning is
         necessary in many nursing functions, such as
         formulating a plan of care. But we don't think
         enough about the meaning of nursing care, and we
         don't realize that one way to care about nursing is to
         think about it. Also, we don't recognize that
         thinking with patients about the meaning of
         proposed treatment and care is caring for them.

Jack: The tendency to think of thought as abstract and
         divorced from concrete and practical affairs is not
         limited to nurses. It is a general tendency in our
         culture. James challenged this misconception by
         asserting that the good life comes from being
         concretely and practically called by visions of a
         better life. He rejected both idealistic visions of the
         good life divorced from practical reality and so-
         called "realistic" approaches to a life that eliminated
         visions of the good. He believed that we are called to

care by people actually making demands on us, and by seeing possibilities for a better life in the events we are involved in.

Anne: In the parable of the Good Samaritan, the Samaritan is called to care by the plight of the injured man. The Samaritan's compassionate response is an example of what Noddings calls natural caring. It also discloses the meaning of integral care in that the meaning of neighborly care, the call to care, and the actual nursing care are all integrally related to each other.

Jack: It is a powerful disclosure of the meaning of being called to nursing care, even though Jesus originally told the parable to disclose the meaning of being a good neighbor as required by a religious commandment. I wonder if our omission of the religious context will disturb the faithful.

Anne: I would think that the faithful would be more concerned about our failure to treat religious ethics in our book. For many nurses, moral commitment involves religious faith.

Jack: I am glad you put it that way. I believe, as did my professor of Christian ethics, that an ethics should stand on its own without requiring religious faith. He did insist, however, that the religious implication of the ethics be considered.

Anne: Surely you are not proposing that we treat the religious implications of our nursing ethics in the conclusion of our book.

Jack: No, but I can indicate how a religious person might interpret our nursing ethics with a little help from Schweitzer. He not only believed that good fortune obligates all human beings, but that God calls the faithful to care for others, especially for the unfortunate. In current theological language, this call is spoken of as ministering to the world, to distinguish it from ministry to a particular religious group.

Anne: The Good Samaritan ministered to the world. He did not ask if the injured man was a fellow

Samaritan before he responded to his plight with
compassionate nursing care.

Jack: Being called by God to minister to the world can
readily incorporate our nursing ethics into the
Jewish, Christian and probably other faiths, even
though our ethics can and does stand on its own.

Anne: Pellegrino's interpretation of profession can also
speak both to those who profess a religious faith and
to those who do not. For Pellegrino, the meaning of
being a professional is professing to use skill and
knowledge to care for the well-being of clients. That
profession is a moral imperative for all
professionals. Religious professionals, however,
could interpret it as a practical profession of faith.

Jack: Does Pellegrino's interpretation of profession mean
that nurses are not professionals if they merely enter
nursing as a job and are proficient in the knowledge
and skills of nursing?

Anne: I can answer that from my own experience. I don't
believe that I entered nursing as a call to care. I was
very much like Lashley, who initially entered
nursing as a job not a calling. Like Lashley, I was
called to care by engaging in the practice of nursing
with its inherent moral sense. I have come to believe
that nurses are continually called to care for
particular patients in different situations by their
plight and by the moral sense inherent in nursing
care. Most nurses do act from a call to care, they just
don't recognize or articulate their care in that way.

Jack: Philosophers could help nurses recognize and
articulate the moral sense of nursing.

Anne: I not only want nurses to recognize the moral sense
of their practice, but to respond to that recognition
by good patient care. Such themes as the meaning of
being a good nurse, caring presence, called to care,
and therapeutic ethics concern nurses acting and
entering into relationships that help others. These
themes may not be considered *real* ethics in some
philosophical circles, but I believe that exploring

these themes is valuable to nurses who are attempting to fulfill the moral sense of nursing practice.

Jack: Ethical considerations can issue calls to care, but not as forcefully as concrete examples. Patients like Midori would call even a narrowly technical and professional nurse into caring, and Beverly's response to Midori would call nurses into sensitive and deep relationships of caring co-presence.

Anne: Is it adequate to just answer the call to care inherent in nursing practice? Doesn't the call to care need to be grounded in an interpretation of the meaning of being human? Notice, I said "grounded" and not "founded," so let's not get into the whole post-modern question.

Jack: Werner Marx (1992) makes a post-modern move in his attempt to reestablish the centrality of compassion in ethics without resorting to traditional Greek metaphysical and Judeo-Christian foundations.

Anne: I've noticed that you often speak of roots rather than foundations. Is that because you want to remain rooted in the Greek and Judeo-Christian traditions, but without being committed to the foundational approach?

Jack: In a certain sense that's true, but I took the term "roots" from Heidegger (1962). Some of his students used to say that Heidegger had roots instead of toes. Seriously, the term "roots" is appropriate for Heidegger's interpretation of human being as being-in-time. Heidegger was challenging modern ratio-nalism that grew out of the Greek contention that the world was founded on logos, an atemporal rational order that was eternal. In contending that we were beings in time, Heidegger was rejecting traditional logos thinking. We did that when we eliminated THE GOOD NURSE from the second chapter and instead treated being a good nurse as fulfilling the moral sense of nursing that has grown out of an ongoing nursing tradition.

Anne: That moral sense does call us to care. I'm glad we
           got rid of the earlier title for Chapter 2, "The Good
           Nurse."

Jack: "The good nurse" sounds like we're seeking Plato's
           ideal form of The Nurse. Unfortunately, the reaction
           against this form of idealism has been so strong that
           it obscures the value of trying to grasp the meaning
           of being good. Taylor (1991) is right when he says
           that being authentic is vacuous if it means no more
           than being able to choose autonomously this or that
           course of action, without some claim to be fostering
           the good. Speaking of being a good nurse—either in
           the sense of being an excellent practitioner or a
           morally good person—makes no sense without
           understanding the meaning of and commitment to
           being a good nurse.

Anne: When we talk of the moral sense, almost
           immediately people challenge us by saying, "How
           do we know what *the* moral sense is, in this day of
           cultural relativity and ethnicity?"

Jack: We can't absolutely know, in this post-modern era
           in which our traditional foundations have been cut
           out from under us. However, I find Taylor (1991)
           informative when he says that striving to be
           authentic makes no sense apart from being able to
           make significant moral judgments. Likewise,
           nursing as practiced makes no sense apart from its
           moral sense.

Anne: If this book has helped nurses recognize the moral
           sense and become committed to it, I will be satisfied.
           However, I don't believe that will satisfy those
           critics who keep pressing us for *the* foundation of
           nursing ethics.

Jack: Those nurses who say it doesn't make sense to talk
           about the moral sense in a time when we are
           confused about foundations continue to make moral
           judgments in their practice—judgments that
           presuppose that nursing has a moral sense. Benner,
           Chinn, Gilligan, Noddings, Zaner, Marx, Taylor,
           Schweitzer, Pellegrino, and James issue a call to care
           that does not require traditional foundations.

A Therapeutic Ethics

Anne: Since nursing has a moral sense that is inherent and primary, it makes sense to talk about nursing ethics as therapeutic. The moral sense of nursing means fostering the well-being of clients, and that also is the meaning of therapeutic.

Jack: We need to distinguish ethical therapy from general nursing therapy, however. Fostering the well-being of the client with a shot of penicillin is different from doing it by ethical considerations.

Anne: But nurses work in both ways and, as we have said, both are integrally related to each other.

Jack: They can, however, be distinguished from each other. For example, you are always telling me about why it is necessary to turn persons in the right way so that they won't get bed sores. That doesn't strike me as ethical therapy, even though by doing it right you are fostering the patient's well-being.

Anne: I thought that we just wrote a whole book trying to help nurses see how their everyday practice involves ethical considerations, not just resolving the big moral questions that usually are treated in traditional nursing ethics books.

Jack: We did. But let me try to further clarify the distinction between ethical therapy and general therapy by considering the case of Tom, even though it's a medical case. Questions such as whether a dialysis machine can make Tom's continued living possible, how long he can live on dialysis, and how often he will have to have dialysis concern medical therapy. But considering what will make Tom's life worth living under the conditions imposed by dialysis, given all of Tom's other problems, strikes me as ethical therapy. That's what Zaner gets Tom to consider.

Anne: Almost any nurse could have engaged in therapeutic ethics by helping Tom consider the implications of dialysis for his life project.

Jack: Of course. When nurses or physicians help patients understand how medical or nursing therapy relates to their life plans or projects, nurses and physicians are engaged in therapeutic ethics.

Anne: So when Tom's physicians are prescribing and giving dialysis, they are fostering the moral sense of health care. But they are doing so by engaging in medical therapy, not therapeutic ethics.

Jack: Yes! I believe I am competent to engage in therapeutic ethics, but it's inconceivable that I could engage in medical or nursing therapy. If I did engage in ethical considerations that were therapeutic, they would be part *of* nursing therapy rather than apart *from* therapy.

Anne: Let's examine some examples of ethical considerations that are *a part of* nursing therapy rather than *apart from* it. In the previous chapter, all of the examples disclose the meaning of therapeutic ethics—Tom, Mrs. French, Lara, Barbara's patient, and Mr. Jones.

Jack: Remember how Cucci helped Mr. Jones learn to relive the body that he was so alienated from and afraid of. Mr. Jones seemed like an entirely different person when he returned to the unit and swept up his nurse and hugged her. He fulfilled the role of one-cared-for, as Noddings interprets it, both in expressing his appreciation for care given and by demonstrating his engagement in the human project of living well in the world. Cucci became his advocate both by helping him determine the meaning of his illness and treatment for his life, and by helping persuade his physicians to turn off the machine and try another form of therapy.

Anne: We nurses have talked so much about advocacy that most nurses will readily understand that being a patient's advocate means engaging in therapeutic ethics. But I believe that therapeutic ethics includes more than advocacy as it is usually understood in nursing. For example, Cucci is engaging in therapeutic ethics by reminding Mr. Jones of his wife's faithful support. Directing him to his relationship with his wife helps him realize that continuing their relationship makes undergoing painful therapy worth it. This is similar to Zaner's helping Tom recognize the value of his work, which led Tom to undergo dialysis. Both cases concerned helping patients discover what makes painful and trying treatment worth suffering through.

Jack: But Lara did not have the option of undergoing difficult treatment that would save her life. She had so much to live for and so little time. Her nurses engaged in therapeutic ethics by helping her live as well as possible during her final days.

Anne: Barbara's patient faced a different problem. He had lost everything that made his life worth living, but he was able to continue living. Barbara engaged in therapeutic ethics by getting down on his level and befriending him. Susan and Zaner helped Mrs. French to choose her own future treatment.

Jack: I think we have made our case that ethics can be therapeutic. But do we want to argue that health care ethics itself is a therapeutic ethics?

Anne: Well, I believe that we should leave that issue to health care ethicists, like Zaner, who are better prepared than we are to deal with it. Let's focus on something more manageable, namely, the value of therapeutic ethics in nursing ethics.

Jack: Okay, but we need to further clarify the meaning of therapeutic ethics. We can do so by describing a way of viewing the relationship of ethics and therapy that is quite different from ours. That way assumes that therapy is primarily concerned with technology and biology. In this therapy, when physicians and nurses encounter moral problems, they call in the expert—an ethicist—to solve the moral problems.

Anne: This implies that medical and nursing therapy is one thing and ethics is another. Therapy creates moral problems, and outsiders, usually educated in philosophy or theology, are brought in to solve problems raised in medical or nursing therapy. But don't those who hold this position believe that the ethical problems are related to therapy?

Jack: The question is, how are they related? Are they adjunct issues to the therapy itself, or are they a vital part of the therapy?

Anne: Haven't we argued throughout our book that, in nursing, ethics and therapy can't be separated in practice?

Jack: Yes. We began with the contention that nursing is a practice with the inherent moral sense of fostering the well-being of clients. Then we said that ethics is concerned with reflexively exploring how well that moral purpose is being fulfilled. Such exploration requires that nursing practice constantly undergo self-criticism, concerning both how the good is achieved and what the good should be. Since nursing is primarily constituted by a moral sense, then it is different from human activities that lack a moral sense. For example, in business, where the dominant purpose is making a profit, ethics considers what is permissible in pursuing that end. Thus, ethics is an adjunct consideration to business's primary purpose—making profit.

Anne: Nursing, unlike business, does have an inherent moral sense and, for this reason, moral concerns cannot be adjunct to nursing practice. But I do not see why recognition of the moral sense *necessarily* makes nursing ethics therapeutic.

Jack: It doesn't, if therapy is limited to restoring the efficient functioning of the body understood as an anatomical machine. For example, a physician who regards a human being as a body and the body as a machine could say that by prescribing a drug, performing an operation, or hooking the body up to a machine, he/she is fostering the patient's well-being and therefore is fulfilling the moral sense of health care.

Anne: Few nurses would reduce the patient's well-being to the efficient functioning of the body understood as a machine. We care for the whole person, not just an efficiently functioning anatomical machine.

Jack: Let's further consider the implications for health care of caring for the whole person, by examining another hypothetical example from medicine. A physician who believes that the anatomical body and the person are one decides that a basketball player needs an operation to ensure the efficient functioning of her body. This operation will prevent her from playing pro basketball. The basketball player says, "No way!" The physician complains that his damn patient doesn't know what's good for her and calls in an ethicist. How would most nurses differ with this interpretation of the relationship of ethics to therapy?

Anne: Most nurses do not think that a human being and the anatomical body are the same. In the case you gave me, the physician is calling in the ethicist to rid himself of a nuisance question that is not, for him, a therapeutic issue. For him the issue is clear—the patient ought to have the surgery because it will improve the functioning of the body. But if we care for the whole person, we should relate her care to her life project. Frankly, I've never read anything in nursing literature that does not assume that consideration of life project, values, and moral commitment are integral aspects of nursing care.

Jack: If nursing therapy is concerned with life projects, and nursing ethics is concerned with how these projects relate to the nursing care given, then ethical considerations are an integral and necessary aspect of nursing therapy.

Anne: The issue here does not concern differences between nursing and medicine, but whether therapy is to be limited to the anatomical body. Most nurses would never consciously limit therapy to the anatomical body, even though, in practice, that occasionally is all that is involved. For example, if a nurse were called on to give a patient a shot of penicillin for gonorrhea, and the patient wanted the shot, and the physician prescribed the shot, and the patient wasn't allergic to penicillin, then the involvement of ethics in therapy would be minimal.

Jack: I'm not sure it's minimal. It raises a moral issue.
Does a nurse have the responsibility to question the
moral behavior of the patient, especially when that
behavior may injure others?

Anne: I've not raised that question because it's usually not
an issue in nursing practice. In normal nursing
practice a nurse would discuss the dangers to the
patient of unprotected sex, especially with the
advent of AIDS, and the possibility of spreading the
disease to others by not using condoms.

Jack: We have discussed this issue in another context. We
did so in asking why neither Perry nor the physicians discussed with the manic patient the moral
issues involved in his decision not to be treated.
Raising this issue implied that we believe that the
patient should have been given an opportunity to
consider whether his decision was morally right,
rather than having the ethicists or the physicians
make this decision for him. Thus, considering what
is morally right would be integrally involved in
informing consent. Put differently, we believe that
nurses are responsible for helping patients face the
moral meaning of their choices regarding illness and
treatment.

Anne: But the case of Midori is quite different in that she
appears morally sensitive to her choices concerning
her illness and its treatment. She decides not to
undergo surgery that would probably kill her, even
though she prefers dying under anesthesia to dying
by suffocation. She is willing to die of suffocation in
order to live the rest of her life at home with her
family. Beverly supports Midori in her struggle to
reach that decision and empowers her to live with it
and carry it out. Beverly's care is therapeutic ethics
in that her nursing care supports her patient's life
project—a life project that seems personally,
morally, and medically sound.

Concluding Dialogue

Jack: Our book has not been just about therapeutic ethics.
If you remember when we originally proposed this

book, we were going to treat nursing ethics as caring presence.

Anne: That's right. But we could not incorporate the whole of nursing ethics in caring presence. We found it necessary to discuss the meaning of being a good nurse, to consider caring as a moral calling, and, finally, to entertain the possibility of nursing ethics being a therapeutic ethics. Can therapeutic ethics encompass being a good nurse, caring presence, and called to care?

Jack: We've struggled long and hard with the relationships between the major themes of this book. We have been dealing with an ethics of practice focused on the meaning of being a good nurse, an ethics of care that incorporates care as a calling and as caring presence, and a therapeutic ethics in which ethics is an integral aspect of nursing therapy.

Anne: I think that nursing ethics involves practice, caring presence, and therapy. Why make one aspect primary just to satisfy those who think that we should conclude with *the* meaning of nursing ethics?

Jack: Both absolutists and complete relativists want *the* answer. The absolutists want *the* answer required by their philosophical system. The relativists seem to think that if you don't have *the* answer to what constitutes the moral good, then further consideration of ethical matters is irrelevant. Neither is satisfied with *some* answers.

Anne: We do have *some* answers. We know that nursing has an inherent moral sense and that this moral sense is concretely instanced in the practice of nursing care. And we do know that being a morally good nurse requires concern for the well-being of the patient that is expressed in effective, attentive, and skillful nursing care.

Jack: We also know that nursing care is experienced by both nurse and patient as caring presence, that this experience is therapeutic for both, and that it confirms the worth and humanity of each. And we do know that you engage in care as a calling.

Anne: The significance of being called to care is what those who speak of *giving* nursing care miss. Care is not something you give; it is a relationship that you enter into and one that you are called into. Sometimes the calling precedes entering the profession; sometimes it comes from being in the profession. It is evoked by feelings of compassion for patients and by responding to examples of caring by those who are fortunate or have special empowerment.

Jack: It also comes from the desire to be an authentic human being guided by visions of the good. Ethical considerations are therapeutic in that they concern how the life project of each patient probably will be affected by illness and treatment. These considerations concern the relationship of the lived body to self, others, and world.

Anne: It's evident that the practice of nursing itself requires such ethical considerations. But given the unsettled identity of both contemporary nursing and philosophy, and our own limitations, I think that we should leave further considerations of nursing ethics to those younger and more expert than we are.

Jack: I hate to end on that note. It sounds as if we have sold out to the fads of our time—youth and experts are our saviors. When I was a young scholar, we sought wisdom and guidance from elders, from those widely read, and from those with significant experience.

Anne: You are widely read, and I am experienced in nursing. And both of us are old enough to have gained some wisdom. But I will be satisfied if we have encouraged nurses to think more deeply about the moral implications of their practice, and if we have called them to thoughtful care.

Jack: Thoughtful care! Surely you're not offering another possible definition of ethics in the conclusion of our book!

Anne: "Thoughtful Care" might be a good title, but I'm merely expressing my hope that our book will evoke thoughtful care by nurses. During my professional life, thought in nursing has primarily concerned how to do this or that, research modeled after science, and applying theories to practice. Only recently have we begun to think about the meaning of nursing. When I said I hoped that we had called nurses to thoughtful care, I was not attempting to introduce a new definition. I merely wanted to assert my conviction that nursing ethics should evoke thinking about concrete practice in ways that help nurses individually and collectively to fulfill the moral sense of nursing.

Jack: Our reflexive dialogue has explored how ethical consideration can contribute to understanding and fulfilling the moral sense of nursing. Nursing ethics helps nurses determine whether their practice individually and collectively lives up to its moral sense, and whether that moral sense is adequate for the challenge of today's world. It also helps nurses recognize and be open to relationships of caring presence that affirm the humanity of patients and support them in their efforts to live well. In addition, ethics helps nurses to hear and answer calls to care given through the moral sense of practice, compassion for others, and a passion for authentic being. Finally, it helps nurses engage in therapy that includes whole persons, their lived bodies in relationship to the world, and their personal projects.

Anne   We have called our interpretation of nursing ethics
and Jack: *Therapeutic Caring Presence,* because the moral sense of nursing is fulfilled through a relationship of caring presence that seeks to foster the well-being of those who are attempting to find and fulfill their projects in the face of illness, debilitation, and treatment. That therapeutic caring relationship is informed and empowered by nursing practice. We hope that our book will call nurses to therapeutic relationships of caring presence, informed and empowered by the practice of nursing.

Study Questions

1. Review Anne and Jack's brief summary of the major themes and the purpose of this book. Which of these themes spoke most forcefully to you as a future or present practicing nurse? Why? What themes did the authors fail to include that you would have included? Why?

2. Why do Anne and Jack believe that Margie is an excellent existential advocate for Mrs. Cooper? Do you agree with their contention that her practice extends the meaning of Gadow's interpretation of existential advocacy? Why or why not?

3. Do you agree with Anne's contention that Margie does not adequately articulate the meaning of advocacy or of the moral sense of nursing? Why or why not? Do you believe that nurses often fail to articulate the moral significance of their care? If so, how can the study of ethics help nurses articulate the moral worth of their practice?

4. Do you believe that Jack is right in describing Margie as a forceful advocate of the moral imperative of nursing, or that Anne is right in describing Margie's care as skillfully maneuvering through a web of connection to persuade others to join her in fulfilling the moral sense of nursing? Why?

5. Why is Jack perplexed over the conflicts between advocates of rights and advocates of care? Do you agree with him? Why or why not?

6. What does Jack believe is the primary struggle in nursing ethics? Do you agree with him? If not, what do you believe the primary struggle is?

7. Describe a "Midori moment" you have experienced. How did it affect you as a nurse and as a person?

8. Anne describes Beverly's care as "so subtle and unobtrusive that its quality is easily unrecognized," especially her use of silence. Give an example of the contribution of these qualities to your patient care.

9. Why does Jack criticize the use of most intervention language in nursing care? Do you agree or disagree with him? Why? Give an example of an inappropriate use of intervention language in nursing. Then, use more appropriate language to describe what was called an intervention.

10. Nurses usually associate caring presence with such hands-on care as bathing. Jack and Anne contend that bathing can be a high level skill developed in the practice of nursing and a way of affirming the worth of patients. Evaluate their contention. Describe other aspects of everyday care in nursing practice that are undervalued as moral activities.

11. Anne and Jack contend that thinking can be a way of caring for patients and for the practice of nursing. Give examples from the book

or from your own experience that support their contention. Do you agree or disagree with their assertion that thinking about the meaning of nursing practice is much neglected in contemporary nursing? Why?

12. Why are Anne and Jack seeking an approach to ethics that is not based on religious or philosophical foundations? How do James, Marx, and Taylor contribute to a nonfoundational approach to nursing ethics?

13. How does Jack distinguish nursing therapy from ethical therapy? Why is Anne disturbed by his distinction? What does Jack mean by his contention that ethical therapy is part of nursing therapy rather than apart from it?

14. Review Anne and Jack's brief interpretation of the cases involving therapeutic ethics. Then choose the one that speaks most forcefully to you. Return to the fuller treatment of the case earlier in the book and interpret the case as an example of therapeutic ethics.

15. Why does Jack believe that whether care involves the whole person or the biological body determines whether or not therapeutic ethics is part of general therapy? Why does Anne believe that this is not an issue in nursing care? Do you agree with Anne? Why or why not?

16. Do you believe that nurses have a moral obligation to help patients consider the moral import of their care and treatment? Why or why not?

References

Gadow, Sally. (1980). Existential Advocacy: Philosophical Foundation of Nursing. In *Nursing: Images and Ideals: Opening Dialogue with the Humanities*, eds. S. F. Spicker and Sally Gadow. New York: Springer.

Harder, Ingegerd. (1993). *The World of the Hospital Nurse: Nurse Patient Interactions—Body Nursing and Health Promotion. Illustrated by Use of a Combined Phenomenological/Grounded Theory Approach*. Aarhus, Danmarks Sygeplejerskehøjskole ved Aarhus Universitet, Skrift-serie fra Danmarks Sygeplejerskehøjskole.

Heidegger, Martin. (1962). *Being and Time*. trans. J. Macquarrie and E. Robinson. New York: Harper and Row.

Marx, Werner. (1992). *Toward a Phenomenological Ethics: Ethos and the Life-World*. Albany, N.Y.: State University of New York Press.

Perry, Clifton B. (1989). The Philosopher as Medical Ethicist: Applying Ethical Theories. In *Philosophers at Work: An Introduction to the Issues and Practical Uses of Philosophy*, ed. E. D. Cohen, 35–42. New York: Holt, Rinehart and Winston.

Ricoeur, Paul. (1977). Phenomenology and the Social Sciences. In *The Annals of Phenomenological Sociology II*, ed. M. Korenbaum, 145–149. Dayton, Ohio: Wright State University.

Taylor, Charles. (1991). *The Ethics of Authenticity*. Cambridge, Mass.: Harvard University Press.

Zaner, Richard M. (1981). *The Context of Self: A Phenomenological Inquiry Using Medicine as a Clue*. Athens, Ohio: Ohio University Press.

Index